Yoga and Childbirth

TONY CRISP

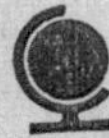

SPHERE BOOKS LIMITED
30/32 Gray's Inn Road, London WC1X 8JL

First published in Great Britain by Thorsons
Publishers Ltd 1975
Copyright © Tony Crisp 1975
First Sphere Books edition 1976
Reprinted 1977

Set in Monotype Times

Printed in Great Britain by
Hunt Barnard Printing Ltd., Aylesbury, Bucks.

Contents

Dedicated To

Ma-Ea, mother of my, and the World's soul.
Betty, mother of my body.
Brenda, mother of my children and my love.
And to mothers everywhere, especially those who
realise that they are not only the mother of their
baby, but also the mother of God.

Introduction

If we were perfect people living in a world made perfect by us, there would be no need for this book. Perhaps all that would be necessary would be to encourage you in your already deeply held convictions. Certainly I would not need to instruct you in them. Your childbirth, like all the other aspects of your life, would arise naturally out of your relationship with life itself.

With most of us this is not the case, and we frequently feel lost and ill-equipped to face even the most basic events of life; so I offer you this book as a guide. I hope it will act as a lantern, however flickering, to give you light in the dark places of your life.

Because we are not perfect people, the book of necessity has to deal with the possible mistakes we may make. Nevertheless, I offer you a method that does work. But a few words of explanation will not be out of place here.

Yoga, in its most integrated forms, takes into account all of a person's nature. Unlike schools of thought which concentrate only on preparing a person's body or thoughts for the business of life's events, yoga works on all levels. Therefore in this book we deal with getting your body, mind and soul ready for the event of childbirth. You may nevertheless argue that I have given a lot of space to mentioning diet. This is so, and for a very good reason. Being the father of five children, and having also taught yoga and relaxation for a number of years, it strikes me time and time again, that women fail to achieve an easy and ecstatic birth as they should, because one or the other aspects of their life have been neglected. There are numerous books on childbirth that teach many of the things mentioned in this book. Most women have already heard about how exercise and relaxation play a part in helping childbirths. But there are virtually no books which explain in adequate detail, how to unite these methods with a proper diet. I mean by this, a diet *specifically* aimed at producing a beautiful baby with an ecstatic birth.

In any case, Christianity is one of the few spiritual disciplines which does not give definite dietary advice. We know of the Jews and their koshered foods, the Hindus and their rules of eating only certain foods and avoiding meat. We know Mohammedans do not touch alcohol or pork. Buddhists are vegetarians. In the ancient yoga books, much was also given about what to eat, how much, and how often. Therefore, the remarks in this book are an integral part of yoga and childbirth. And I know that if the postures alone are practised, without adequate nutrition, the results are not by any means as satisfactory. In other words, the percentage of success is much lower.

1.

Being Movement

Despite having taught yoga postures for a number of years, I nevertheless feel that the best exercise is that which expresses our functions. There is nothing more fulfilling and satisfying than movements in which, and through which, we express our feelings, our longings, our needs and our life. Stop for a moment and consider the hundreds of movements we make each day, whereby we fulfil ourselves, provide our needs, express our feelings and vent our anger. Take some of the most basic movements and postures – going to the toilet, eating, breathing, working to provide our needs, loving each other, holding hands, having a baby.

Without going any further than these few basic movements, let us look at them and see what a wonder of satisfaction or frustration can lie behind them.

Going to the toilet, for instance; what is it all about as a movement? It is obvious in this that we fulfil a need on the part of the body to be rid of waste. In fulfilling this need fully we have a sense of pleasure and satisfaction. Something has triggered off a movement in the muscles of the colon, and if this urge to move is not allowed expression, then this part of our being is not allowed to satisfy itself. In that degree we are unsatisfied.

Similarly, eating requires movements of the body, some gross, some subtle. The way we perform these movements, the quality or poverty of being we bring to this activity, largely controls, once again, the degree of pleasure and satisfaction we harvest from the whole process of eating and digestion. Many people have seen in their own experience that to eat in the relaxed company of friends produces in them quite a different state of digestion and well-being than to eat alone. It is also well known that to eat while emotionally upset very often leads to vomiting, or at least to impoverished digestion and absorption. So it is not only the movement, but the quality, emotional tone, and fullness of expression that we bring to it that largely controls the degree of satisfaction we reap from eating.

In our breathing this is particularly noticeable, as it is a process we can watch more easily. In doing so we can see that our breathing intimately mirrors not only our physical activity, but also the state of our soul. Not only does our breathing quicken or slow as we exert ourselves or rest, but also, while sitting reading a book, or when absorbed in a play, our breathing reflects our emotional state, either being long and slow in peace, or agitated in emotional turbulence. So much is this so that psychological problems can literally be diagnosed by an examination of one's breathing.

Work should be fulfilling
When we come to the movements we make in our work, in a general sense, the man or woman who works hours in a garden, planting and hoeing, to grow food to fulfil their needs, is having a far more fulfilling exercise than a person who goes to a gymnasium simply to 'get enough exercise'.

This undoubtedly needs further comment lest it be misunderstood. I am not saying that the gardener will be healthier, stronger, or more exercised. I am saying that in general there will be more satisfaction and fulfilment in it when there is a direct connection between a fulfilment of a need or love, and the activity performed. If the person in question sees that the produce grown fulfils the need for food; if he likes this form of activity and is also expressing his sense of pleasure; if he is also intellectually interested in the technical side of the garden – then he is literally fulfilling himself in innumerable ways. Not only does he use his physical energy to provide for his physical needs, but in doing so he experiences pleasure, satisfies the need of the mind to occupy itself in learning, study and application; and besides all this, the need for fresh air and sunlight is fulfilled; and possibly in some cases, especially in flower gardening, his sense of beauty also.

Obviously I have used gardening merely as an example. What I am trying to emphasise is the need, in our activities, to satisfy ourselves as fully as we can. If we do not recognise our needs then we may easily overlook them and feel incomplete. If we do not find activities which satisfy several parts of our being in the one action, as in the above example, then we may either be rushing around trying to fit in innumerable different activities to satisfy different needs, or remain largely frustrated.

We can see more of these needs in the act of love, and its movements; or just in cuddling. Likewise, the birth of the baby expresses definite movements, a reflection of Life itself.

We can therefore begin to see that our life is largely a matter of being ourselves as fully as we can, and in this, finding the reward of pleasure and satisfaction. Having a baby falls into a similar category. Margaret Brady, in her book *Having a Baby Easily*, says, 'It is a CREATIVE function. It is an ATHLETIC function. It is a SPIRITUAL function.' This is a very helpful definition, because it aids us to see that, being an 'athletic' function, or at least involving as it does muscular activity of a strenuous kind, it therefore requires the mother to be capable of such activity.

I do feel, however, that this definition may make us overlook the fact that in being a mother it is not just *parts* of our life that are involved. Really, our whole being is involved, from heights to depths – body, soul, and spirit. This is why I believe yoga has such a lot to teach us about childbirth. But Margaret Brady is certainly right when she says, 'Since it is also an ATHLETIC function, she must have the NECESSARY ATHLETIC TRAINING for the event.' But, as we have seen, the quality and fulfilment of this 'athletic event' is conditioned by the emotions we bring to bear on it; our intellectual interest and involvement, which is shown in the very act of reading this book; our relationship with our source of life, and the way we link up our other interests with pregnancy.

Movement is essential to life
Looking at exercise from a slightly different viewpoint, the medical or physiological, we can see that movement is essential to life. In fact, movement is the very expression of life. One of the most obvious differences between the living and the dead is movement, for while we live, movement never ceases. Whereas machines wear out through use, the body literally thrives on being made to exercise its systems and possibilities. It comes to the peak of its efficiency through being used. This is so obvious to us that it needs no argument. Our joints become stiff with inactivity, supple with use; our muscles small and flabby with disuse, large and sleek with activity. Great activity and deep relaxation are laws of the universe, as well as of our body.

Recent research has proved that much of what we call ageing is due not to 'natural' processes, but to lack of correct nutrition, exercise and rest. People like Hauser, Kordel and Bragg are proof of their own philosophy in regard to diet, exercise and rest. They are all 'elderly', but each has little or no sign of ageing. Modern medical research has uncovered many of the processes which cause this, but in general the inadequacy of diet and exercise can be summed up in its results by seeing what it does to our bones. Bones are not dead structures, but are made of living bone cells, called osteocytes. As in all other cellular structures, there is a continuous process of breakdown and repair. In many people, especially in the aged, the process of building up does not keep pace with the process of breakdown. This produces weak, fragile bones. One often hears of old people falling and breaking a thigh or hip. In fact, what usually happens is that the bone has become so weakened it has broken and caused them to fall. It is now realised that such fragility in the bones is not a process of age but is due to the lack of sex hormones in the blood and inadequate exercise. The sex hormones stimulate production of osteocytes. Similarly, muscular activity puts strains on the skeleton, and this stimulates not only the flow of blood but also the production of bone cells. These bone cells use proteins, calcium salts, and vitamins C and D in building fresh 'bone'. Thus it becomes obvious that lack of sufficient exercise and nutrients can cause degenerative changes in the body. The degeneration of the bones is but one example of such changes throughout the whole body.

Exercise during pregnancy
There is, in the minds of many people, an opposing force to this idea of exercise during childbirth. This undoubtedly springs from the time when any pregnant woman was looked upon as a delicate and sick person. In many cases the women went to bed and stayed there throughout pregnancy. Any activity or stretching was thought to be dangerous to mother and child. We can certainly sympathise with this attitude because, after all, due to the way of life at that time, pregnancy *was* dangerous. Mothers and babies so frequently died that such excessive care can be seen as an attempt to avoid any stress or strain. Yet really, the lack of a certain amount of stress and strain is in itself weakening. Not only do animals which have been sheltered from a healthy amount of stress easily die of shock, but the same is true of humans.

To balance this somewhat, we have to realise that during pregnancy there may be a much greater tendency to tiredness. Or to put it another way, there may be a need for more frequent rests. If such tiredness arises, first of all ask yourself whether sufficient protein is being taken, but in all cases give way to the desire for rest. The energy level throughout the day can be enormously increased by taking a breakfast rich in protein, with some carbohydrates, fats, and sugar.

This brings us to the point where we must consider the actual exercises that will be most beneficial. Such exercises must have three aims in view. One is to stimulate all the body activities and thus promote healthy activity and stress in the body. The second aim is to strengthen and prepare the particular muscles that will be used during the actual birth. The third aim is to make the body and personality capable of satisfying movement. This needs some further explanation. But rather than attempt to explain this intellectually with words, I will do it through the use of the postures as they are given.

Interest and Stimulus of Exercise

As we have already seen, for general health the muscles, bones, organs and the systems, such as circulation, nervous, lymphatic and respiratory, need to be used and stimulated. We can see this response of the body to use in watching how muscles respond to exercise. When all the materials of nutrition are supplied there arises a tremendous satisfaction from muscular effort, especially when directed towards some goal or aim. In such circumstances, the muscles respond to the stress imposed on them by becoming larger, beautifully shaped, sleek and responsive.

We can see all this in the lovely bodies of most ice skaters and athletes. Therefore, if you already get very frequent exercise in an activity you thoroughly enjoy, such as swimming, skating, walking, gardening, riding, etc., then your general needs are most likely fulfilled. But so few of us actually call upon our bodies enough to really perspire, and make the heart pump and the breath rush in and out in deep inhalations, and this is what is needed frequently each week.

Even when such demands are made upon our body, how often do we look upon the exertion as a pleasure? In most cases it is felt as a burden, a troublesome task to be got over with as quickly as possible in order to sit down and swallow yet more tea or coffee, or inhale nicotine. When our body is healthy, as it soon should be if the dietary programme is followed, exercise becomes such a joy that one often literally seeks it out for the pleasure of doing it. In other cases, the tired, jaded feeling that makes one shy away from exercise, is literally wiped away by doing the very thing avoided.

In so many yoga classes people have come to me afterwards and said, 'You know, I nearly gave it a miss tonight because I had such a headache and felt so tired. But while I

was doing the postures it all seemed to go, and now I feel fine.'
I believe this applies to many forms of exercise because of
the interest and stimulus they provide.

In approaching these exercises and postures, we must try
to express some of the principles mentioned at the beginning
of this chapter. They must not be approached as if they were
a task or discipline one has *got* to perform. Neither should
they be entered into as a thing to be got over as quickly as
possible, or with too much aggressiveness and haste, so that
you do damage to yourself. They should be approached in
the same way the potter approaches his clay, or the gardener
his garden, or a sculptor his stone. That is, with a recognition
that energy is going to be expended, but with an end in view,
and as a creative activity which will also fulfil our needs.
Nearly everybody performs best if an ideal, a goal, or an aim
spurs them on. Working for nothing soon gets boring. But if
the work promises a reward of some kind, then we can
direct our energy into it far more fully and gain much satisfaction. Therefore, even before we begin, we must have a very
clear idea of what we are aiming at, and what we hope to
achieve. This alone can turn a task or regime into a pleasure.
Therefore, hold in mind the goal of an easy birth, and producing a beautiful baby. Realise that your exercises are
shaping your baby's body just as they shape your own.

A pattern of exercises

The following pattern of exercises is written in a way that
attempts to incorporate these ideas and benefits. They include
both general and particular exercises, and through bringing
thoughtfulness, and the goal of a beautiful baby easily born,
to the postures, we enhance their value. The exercises should
be performed, whenever possible, some time after a meal, in
a well ventilated but not draughty room, or out-doors in the
sun if you are lucky. Your clothing should be loose and light,
and you should have a blanket on the floor to sit or lie on.
Four to five times per week is sufficient, but you can perform
these exercises daily if you enjoy them. Having sorted out
time and place, let us begin.

In practising yoga to attain an easier and more joyful childbirth, we have to learn how to relate to our body. As the uterine movements to expel the baby are an expression of Life's processes, we have to learn how to co-operate with Life in bringing forth our baby.

1. *Circles of protection.* Stand in the centre of your blanket and imagine an invisible sphere around you, above and beneath, so you are in the centre of it. All the world is shut out, and the irritations of one's affairs cannot break through this invisible protection. Realise as you imagine this invisible protection that your baby, too, is in just such a circle of protection; in fact, many circles of protection. First the water within the membrane protects, bathes and acts as a buffer against pressure, knocks and harm. Then your uterus surrounds this, holding the baby firm and steady in your love. Around this is your body, which protects the baby by surrendering its nourishment and strength, a circle of goodness and health within which the baby can flourish. Interpenetrating these circles of protection are your emotions and thoughts in which the baby is immersed, just as truly as he is immersed in the inner fluid. Therefore, as you stand within your sphere of protection, look at your emotions and thoughts, to see what you have brought with you.

But first, imagine that from the top of the sphere a rope dangles and is attached to the very top of your head. From this you are firmly suspended, hanging in the middle of your sphere. Imagine your head growing up and up, very gently, so that the spine and body straighten without effort, and all the parts of your body are coming into perfect shape and condition. Now look to see if you are holding on to any distressing emotions such as worry, fear, dislike or envy. Let go of them as if you literally had hold of them with your hands. Do this by opening the hands and completely relaxing. Take your time over this. There is no hurry, and although it may at first seem difficult, you will soon manage it. You can use your own ideas or methods to achieve the same end, of relaxation of mind and emotions within the image of a beautiful and healthy body.

Now imagine that the rope goes right through your body to your feet. But instead of a rope, see it as a column of light. Imagine as clearly as you can this column of light radiating to every part of your – and the baby's – being. Melt into the light as if it were a healing force reaching every part of you.

2. *An expression of energy.* The reason such images as the sphere, rope and light are used is because in yoga it is realised that one's thoughts and emotions play a large part in shaping your body. This is so obvious we often overlook it; but when we feel depressed or angry, our expression and posture are quite different from when we feel gay or loving. When a particular attitude of thought or emotion is held for a long time, it literally shapes our facial expression and our posture. Also, no matter what our conception of the reason for our existence is, something causes us to be. Whether that something is chemical, biological, cosmic, or divine, yet we exist, and have been created. We symbolise this creative something as the column of light, which fills our body. This is done because so often our conscious attitudes and activities may put us out of harmony with the creative force of which we are an expression. This imagining in some degree helps us release the creative energies again, instead of blocking them as we may have been doing.

As everything we do is an expression of this energy or 'something' which we are, we will use this image throughout. For instance, electricity can be expressed as heat, light, power, sound, and so on. Likewise, this energy filling our body can be expressed, first as the characteristics of life, such as movement, awareness, feelings, memory, digestion, and so on; but also as speech, thought, love, and the other human activities, which express it in a multitude of ways. In our exercises we are going to do it consciously instead of unconsciously as we usually do. For instance, every time we speak we are expending or directing our energy into sound. In the exercises we are going to direct it in other ways.

Relate to your body
Before going on to the other postures, let us begin to learn

how to relate to our body. Lie on your back on your blanket, breathing deeply. Then, after a few breaths breathe in deeply and hold it for as long as possible. I mean really struggle to hold your breath.

There is a world of difference between just reading something and actually doing it. Therefore, even if on reading what I have to say you think you have got the idea, this is not enough. Childbirth is not an intellectual affair. It confronts you with the fantastic powers of your body. If you relate to them poorly, then you may get knocked about in the process. So, apart from needing to be fed in the right way, we also need to relate to it correctly. This is what we are doing.

You will obviously find that after a short time of holding your breath you begin to become uncomfortable. If you persist, the discomfort turns into a struggle. Beyond that lies pain and convulsions. Further still – blackout. This practice can be discontinued as soon as you clearly see how you relate to your body.

So, what does all this prove? Well, first of all that we can interfere wth the spontaneous processes of our being. Our conscious will can interfere with the life forces that cause us to exist. Therefore, we, as a conscious person, can co-operate with or go against that which causes us to exist. We find, however, that interference causes discomfort – pain – blackout. If we only half interfered, we could do so for days, and the sequence might not quickly escalate to pain. Instead we would exist in continuous discomfort of body and mind.

Childbirth is also a spontaneous process like breathing. We have a similar relationship with it. Therefore, how can we co-operate instead of interfere?

3. *Tension.* Let us try another test to further define this. Lie on your blanket face up. Tense your whole body fairly hard. Tense: legs – hips by tensing the rectum – shoulders by pulling them up to the ears – arms by clenching the fists – mouth by clenching the teeth – face by wrinkling the forehead. Become aware of how this tension feels by passing your awareness over your body. Then slowly relax, noticing the feeling of dropping tension. Do this twice more, particularly

noticing how the tension restricts breathing and in fact all spontaneous movements. The dropping of tension frees the body to move easily. Only go this far for the first two weeks of your practice. Use the following methods in subsequent weeks. In the first two weeks, pass on to the other postures. That is, carry on with No. 4.

Second two weeks. You need a partner for this, husband or friend. Lie on your blanket. Tense and relax a few times to get the feel of letting go of your body. Then, become *as limp as possible*. Your partner now takes an arm and moves it gently in various changing directions, and then the other arm and legs. You or your partner may notice that even though you 'let go', nevertheless the arms or legs are not really relaxed. Either you try to help perform the movement instead of being limp, or the muscles tense up quite by themselves. If they do not, then you are doing very well. In any case, practise this with your partner. If you have to do your postures alone, then you can save this practice until a time when you have help. But your husband might enjoy doing this and the postures with you, so do them together if at all possible. Or else advertise in your local paper for another 'mum' who wishes to do yoga relaxation with you.

Third two weeks. The same as above, but while the arms or legs are being moved, tense them slightly and then let go again. This conscious tensing helps you to become aware of remaining tense areas, and how to let go of them. The whole practice is getting you used to being 'moved' and relaxing into the movement.

Fourth two weeks. The same as above for a shorter period, then turn over on to your side or front, depending on the size of your 'bump'. Kneeling beside you, your partner should, with slightly cupped hands, gently slap you all over shoulders, back, hips and legs. Let yourself go into the pleasure of it. If your partner does not do it as well as you feel he or she could, explain how (harder, softer, longer, quicker, slower) he or she can make it more enjoyable for you. This slapping is very relaxing, and so rest in the position for a while afterwards. Five minutes is long enough for the slapping. After these two weeks the practice can be carried on throughout pregnancy – or discontinued if a partner is hard to come by.

4. *Squatting*. One of the things I find very beautiful in animals is their characteristic postures. I have watched robin hens, during their mating ritual, take up the posture of a tiny fledgling, with mouth wide open and eager. The robin cock, as an expression of his love, collects all the choicest titbits, and feeds her as if she were a baby. Dogs have their characteristic pose for their toilet, the male cocking one leg, the female squatting. Such postures are quite instinctive, and

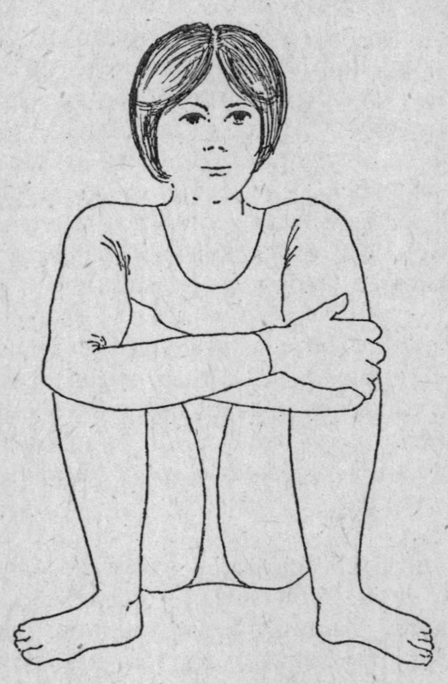

1. The Squat. Recommended as an excercise for childbirth.

to use them fulfils the deepest feelings or drives of the animal. Human beings also have such 'natural' postures, but so few of us are in harmony with our deepest feelings that we usually have nothing but a perverted instinctive drive, or one that is in many ways sick. I later mention one of these characteristic postures in giving details of Dr Wilhelm Reich's researches into the sexual act. Alexander, and the technique he developed, also demonstrate that there is an instinctive spinal posture which if destroyed by tensions, fears, inhibitions, can cause much ill-health. This links very directly to the findings of Reich, who similarly found that the 'destroyed' sexual posture led to dissatisfaction and illness.

The squatting posture that follows is mankind's instinctive toilet posture. It also stretches naturally the genital areas that will be stretched in childbirth. It keeps these parts healthy through exercise and the increased flow of blood and nutrition to the area. Women in some races, such as the Eskimos, are said to actually give birth to their children in this position. It would seem to be the best position where the birth is quick and easy. This position can actually be simulated during birth if you wish, by having plenty of cushions behind you as you lie on your back. Then grasp the legs behind the knees, bringing the legs up and head forward, thus simulating the posture. If at all possible, by all means actually squat while giving birth to your baby. For our fifth baby, my wife used this posture and found it far easier than lying on the back. This should only be used during the bearing-down phase, however.

It is also an advantage, wherever possible, to actually use this posture when going to the toilet. It is certainly the most hygienic method, as one never has to sit on the seat, but lift it and stand on the toilet rim. It also places far less strain on the inner organs during defecation. But even the practice of this posture will help prepare the muscles for childbirth. If you find that your heels will not touch the floor when you squat, then use a fairly thick book to place under the heels, and make balance easier.

Start by standing upright, keeping the eyes fixed on a

particular point to aid balance. Squat down not too fast, breathing in as you do so. Now come up again breathing out as you rise. Repeat this at least ten times straight off, paying particular attention to the deep regular breathing. If you find you can do ten easily, then go on for thirty, fifty, or more. The aim is to stimulate the circulation, perspiration and heart-beat, but particularly the breathing. Hold the idea in the mind of the blood flushing each part of the body, carrying away rubbish, and supplying nourishment and oxygen to each cell. Do this exercise with the express purpose of achieving this, and keeping the muscles healthy and strong. Before beginning this, take several breaths in level one breathing. (A description of breathing levels is given in chapter 4.) As you begin, change into level two, and if necessary, level three. Make sure you breathe right out each time. With all breathing, imagine filling the body with the light as you breathe in.

Whether you do this exercise or not, the next part should be done. After doing all the repetitions of squatting up and down, squat down and stay down in the squat position. As mentioned, use a book if necessary. Allow as many muscles as possible to become relaxed and loose. Make your arms comfortable over your knees, or fingers touching the floor to aid balance. Let the head droop in relaxation. Become aware of your body and relax. Close the eyes and feel the pleasant sensations of your body.

5. *Relaxation*. It must be realised that the actual muscles that expel the baby at birth are not those of the abdominal wall. It is the enormous muscles of the uterus, which are not voluntary muscles like those in arms and legs. The muscles of the uterus, in which the baby is encased, are like those of our heart, beyond the influence of our conscious will. Or at least, while we can consciously choose to move an arm, it is much more difficult to make the heart muscles beat faster or slower but it can be done – in fact, we are often doing it. Whenever we are emotionally moved by a film or incident, our heart speeds up its action. We can thus control our heart by directing or changing our moods. All the other involun-

tary muscles are also influenced by our moods. While it may be difficult to actually exercise the muscles of the uterus, we can become more conscious of activity in this area, and thus have more control over it. A tense emotional state results in tension in the muscles surrounding the birth canal, and will make birth more difficult. Therefore, while in the squat position, practise the following.

Close the eyes and relax the whole body. Concentrate your attention on your sexual organs. Be aware of their shape, the pressure of clothes, and any other sensations. Bring your attention inwards to see if you can sense the uterus itself. When the baby is moving, this will of course be easier, as the sensations of movement will help to outline the feeling of the uterus. Take your time over this. Now tense the anus, sexual organs and face. This may be difficult if you have never done it before, but it becomes easy with practice. Tensing the anus for instance is the same tension we make when we wish to go to the toilet badly, but have to wait. The same applies to the genitals, as the two parts usually tense together. Try not to involve the abdominal muscles in this, only the face, genitals and anus. Hold the tension for a few seconds, then *slowly* release it. Now try to tense the abdominal ('stomach') muscles without tensing the face or genitals. Slowly release this, and bring your attention to the face. Nearly all tensions are reflected in our face; we can therefore find a corresponding relaxation throughout the body. So let all expression and tension drop from the face. After a few moments, start again from tensing the genitals, and go through the whole procedure five to six times.

The reason this complicated procedure is suggested is that our body tensions work against each other without our being aware of it. During birth the uterus tenses to eject the baby through the birth canal. Many women, however, unconsciously tense the anus and genitals, thus restricting the birth canal in size. Also, during birth, the abdominal muscles tense to aid the uterus in its work. But again, this tension often involves other muscles that should remain relaxed. Therefore, this little exercise helps you to (*a*) distinguish between abdominal and genital tension, (*b*) tense or relax each separately and thus enable you to relax the genitals during uterine or abdominal contraction, and (*c*) relax the face, and thus relax the whole body between contractions. You must realise, however, that during the first stages of labour you must not aid the contractions of the uterus by pushing, or bearing down with your abdominal muscles. This is because the uterus can be likened to a bottle with the head of the baby at the narrow neck trying to get out. The 'neck' of the uterus must be stretched gradually, which is done by the contractions of the uterus itself. Once the opening is large enough for the baby's head to pass through, then you can bear down. Of course, the nurse will tell you when is the right time, but until then resist every temptation lest you tear the mouth of the uterus slightly.

Each time you go to the toilet to defecate, become very aware of (*a*) the relaxation of the anus, and (*b*) the tension of the abdomen to expel stools. This is exactly the state of affairs we want during the birth, so never fail to go to the toilet *consciously*, so that during birth you can relax anus and genitals during contractions.

6. *Imaginative cuddling*. Now curl up and rest on your blanket, lying on your right side. Curl up as much like a baby as possible, bringing the knees up. Close your eyes and imagine that the *light* is passing through your body in a circle, leaving the top of the head and circling round in front to enter the base of the spine again. Imagine it going slower and slower, and then just see yourself floating in that light which is flooding your whole body. As you float, imagine cuddling your baby, enfolded in your love.

Such imaginings should not be thought of as comforting fantasies. Imagination stimulates emotion, and as you will see in the later chapters, your baby is vitally aware of your emotions. Therefore, if you feel love during this imaginative cuddling, it is no fantasy, the baby will feel it too, which is just as helpful as love during breast-feeding.

The things you have learnt when relaxing arms and legs with your partner's aid, should be applied during the postures.

That is, let go of any tension not required to hold the posture.
7. *The Seed Posture*. Because we are 'Being Movement' rather than just mechanically 'doing' postures or exercises, we will approach the classical yoga postures in a novel way. In most books a picture or drawing of a body position is shown or described, and one then attempts to 'get into' that posture. Sometimes such postures are nigh on impossible for us. To attempt postures in this way is to do them mechanically. We are like machines copying movement which may be quite wrong for us as we are. Our body contorts and strains in an effort to achieve the pose, which is quite alien to the yoga idea of union. To co-operate and work with our body is to express this idea of union, while to mechanically take up a posture is often to deny and impose it.

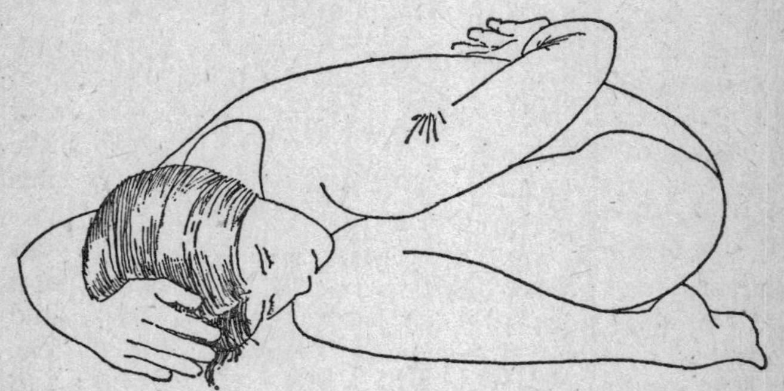

2. The Seed. Lying dormant.

Let us therefore feel our way into doing the postures as means of expression, not repression. One of the loveliest to begin with is the Seed Posture.

Start by holding in mind a dried-up seed. Now experiment with body positions in an attempt to find one which expresses what it might feel like to be such a dried-up seed. Take your time. Move your body around until you inwardly feel *right* as a seed. You might find as you enter into the posture more fully that your arms, legs, or head, or any part of you, does not feel quite expressive enough of the seed you are express-

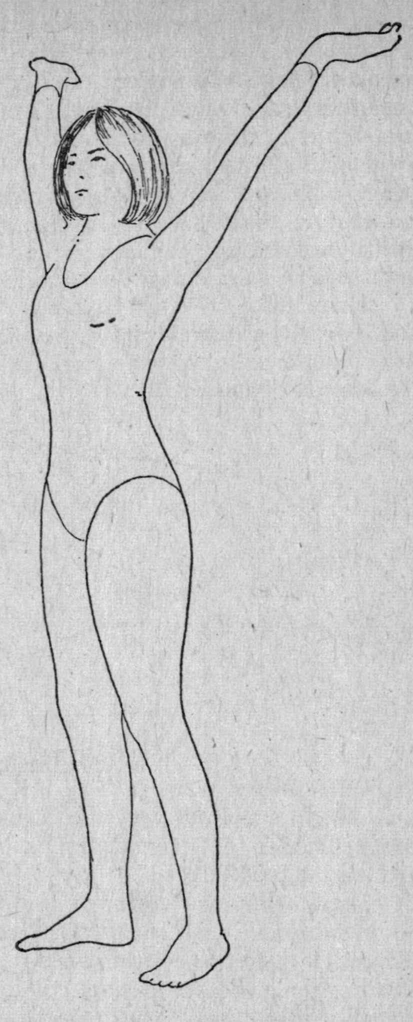

3. The seed—now a plant—opening to the sun.

ing. If so, move until you feel inwardly content with your position.

When you have got this far, turn your attention away from awareness of your body position towards what you feel inside, emotionally or in thought. Ask yourself how a dried seed might feel. Think of it as a tiny focus of Life as yet unexpressed. Does it feel lonely? Does it have a desire to burst open and grow? What is going on inside it? Do not worry about being precise. Let your feelings go where they will, meanwhile maintaining the posture for a minute or so.

The question may now arise in your mind as to what posture *should* you have taken on. There is no answer. You take on any position which feels right to you, and which for you expresses the feeling of being a dried-up seed. This is all we are seeking. This is Being Movement!

8. *The seed grows*. After a minute or so of the seed posture, imagine that, as a seed, you are now in the warm earth, and water penetrates you. You expand, and the sleeping life within you thrusts out and grows. Roots push into the earth, a stem swells and rises to the light.

As you do this, let any movements or positions occur which suggest themselves to you. Let your emotions flow and arise as postures and movements. Open to the light, while holding firmly to the earth. Then let the light penetrate your very being.

Again, no particular postures are being looked for. Kneel, stand, move your arms, your head, lie down, in whatever way comes to you. Don't think it up, let it arise from within you as much as possible.

9. *Be a baby*. Rest from the rigours of growing, and when rested, be a baby crawling. Imagine everything is new to you. You haven't seen things before. You are having a lovely time crawling around, touching things, stumbling maybe, and generally exploring enjoying yourself, and doing whatever comes to you to do as a baby. This includes having a cry, or sucking your thumb, if you bump your head.

10. *Be a lioness*. Again rest, and let the baby mood disappear.

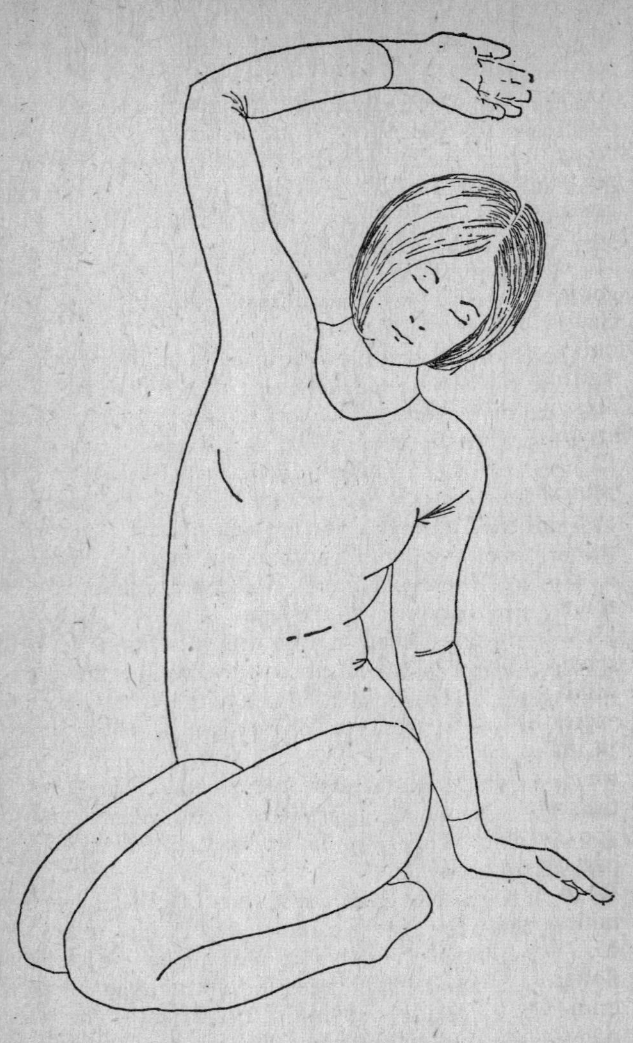

4. The plant growing and putting out leaves.

When it has, let the feeling grow in you of being a lioness sprawled in the sun, full up and without a care in the world. If you like, be a pregnant lioness. If a fly settles on your nose, move your nose like lionesses do. Growl a little if you feel like doing so. Or if somebody has annoyed you during the week, get a cushion and imagine you are a lioness giving them a good bite and a clout with your paws. Having got this out of your system, *then* sprawl out in the sun.

11. *Be a turtle*. When you have sprawled for long enough, and got your breath back from being a baby or an angry lioness, change into a turtle. Imagine the giant shell on your back, into which you can retreat. Find a position which expresses the turtle's stiff, slow legs, and its emerging and withdrawing neck. Hold the position for some time, and then maybe walk around a little, or retreat into your shell.

12. *Be a snake*. Now you are a snake, as flat on the floor as your bump allows, and lifting your head up to look around, or frighten an enemy. Use your hands a little to help, but remember snakes don't have hands to lift their heads, so be a snake as much as possible. Hold the position for a while, and rest.

13. *Be a seagull*. Take on the feelings of a seagull, wings out-spread, not moving, but gliding almost motionless on the wind. Again experiment to find a suitable body position to express this, and hold it as long as is comfortable.

14. *Be an opening flower*. It is night-time. You are a flower which has closed up tightly against the cold and the dew. But the sun is rising warm and calling. Slowly and with gladness you open to the light, and allow it to fall on the very tenderest part of you hidden under layer after layer of beautiful petals. When you are fully open, hold the posture for some time until the feeling of it fades.

15. *The flower dies*. As it fades, life fades in you, and as the flower, your petals begin to fall, and your stem dries up and crumbles to the earth, into which you are absorbed. You are quite dead. Your body has returned to the earth from whence it came. The Life which lifted up the earth into the leaves has withdrawn into its source. But wait; your seeds were formed

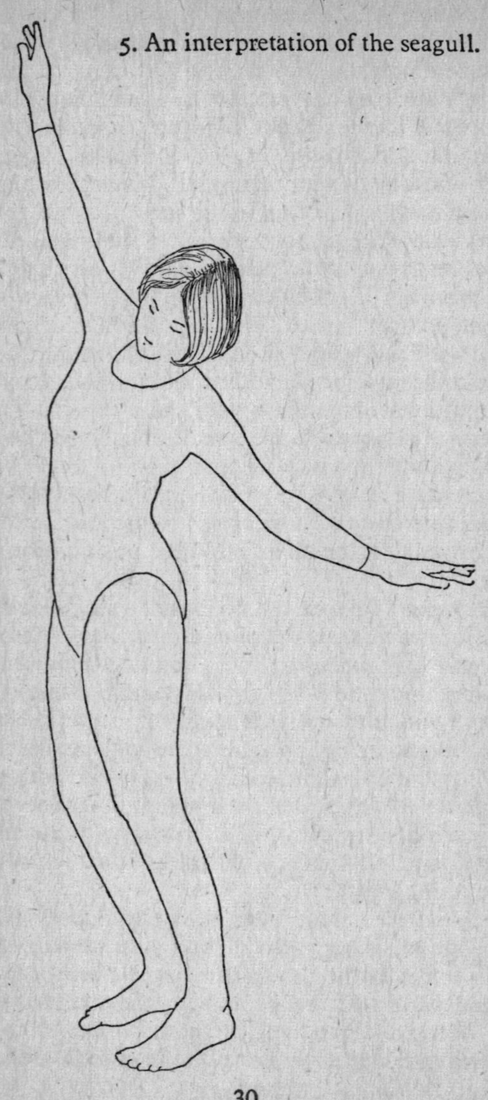

5. An interpretation of the seagull.

as you opened to the sun, and they have dropped into the earth. Your body is the earth, your baby the seed. New life is arising!

16. *Be a holy person.* Now become a holy person, sitting alone but not feeling alone, for you are filled with the realisation that Life fills every cell of your body, and through it you connect with all other living things. There is deep peace in your being. Act out within yourself how it might feel to be such a person. How do they feel within themselves? What expression is on their face? How do they sit? How do they arrange their hands as a posture of how they feel inside? Let it happen to *you*!

Some people find that when they act out these postures and movements, tears of sorrow or joy are released. Or else spontaneous movements begin to occur to them. In a few cases, it is as if they were merely a spectator while Life in them moves their body.

If this happens to you, it is quite safe to allow it to happen, although it may seem strange. But it is no stranger or miraculous than the movements Life is continuously performing with your body. Breathing, eating, digestion, heartbeat, are all movements Life makes spontaneously. Being used to these, we do not feel them as strange. We *expect* them. During birth our body also goes into spontaneous contractions, and again we *expect* this. But inasmuch as we can trustingly go along with such spontaneous movements, to that degree, Life and you can co-operate to give birth to your baby.

The only difficulty occasionally arising is that these spontaneous movements lead to things we might not judge to be good. When we eat something poisonous, Life in us causes us to retch and vomit. This is an unpleasant feeling and experience, but it is Life's way of healing us and protecting us. During our life we may have 'swallowed' many poisonous emotions, desires, thoughts or experiences. When we relax and let Life act on us or flow through us, as in these postures, it sometimes tries to have us 'vomit' up these past poisons. Thus if we lost someone we love, and buried our pain and grief, we may, if we let spontaneous movements or emotions

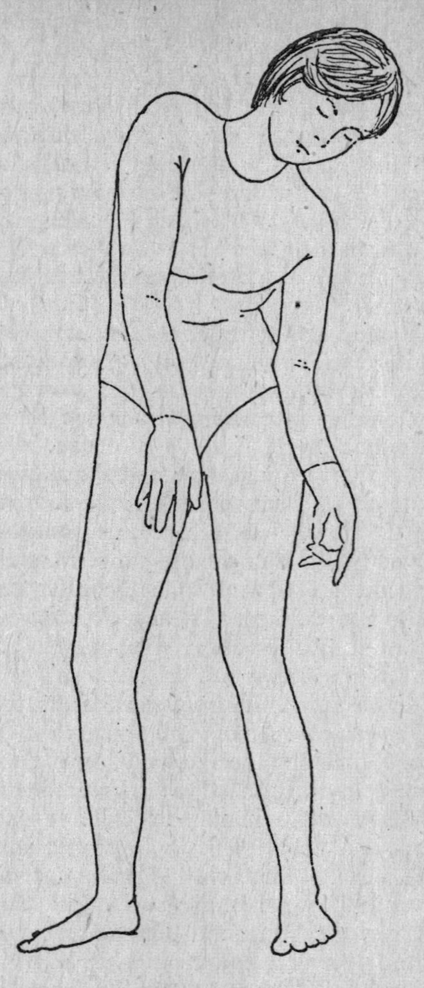

6. After flowering the plant begins to fade.

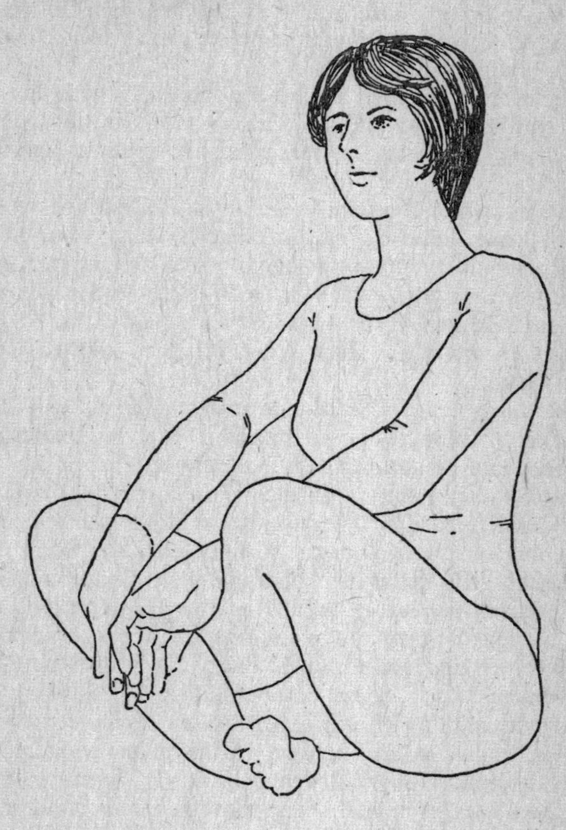

7.'Be a holy person.'

arise, suddenly weep bitterly as this past grief is cleansed out of us. The advantage of this is that such pains and griefs inside us block the natural activity of Life in us. They are one of the main causes we cannot completely relax and experience a fully joyful childbirth.

Therefore, inasmuch as you can, go along with any outpourings. Let them happen. There is no harm in them for your baby, only help. But in fact, very few people experience them.

17. *Be an oyster*. Deep in the sea, oysters silently grow their lovely pearls. Be an oyster, hinged at the waist. Your baby is your pearl, and you are closing your shell around it. As with other postures, hold it until the feeling fades. But as you do it, feel the hard shell formed by legs, trunk and arms. All your life is enclosed by the shell. When you have finished, slowly open again.

18. *Be an earthquake*. Lastly, be an earthquake. Do it in any position you like, lying or standing. Imagine tremendous tensions and pressures slowly building up deep inside you. These are the anger and violence of the earth. Gradually feel them build up, and then maybe just a twitch as the first sign of the enormous release hits the surface. Then the whole earth shakes and vibrates as the wonderful release is accomplished. Let yourself go into it as fully as you are capable. Shout, groan, bang with your arms and legs, roll about, or whatever is in you to do. Don't be held back in any of these 'Being Movements' by a sense of foolishness. These things are tremendously helpful, and we are not just playing for the sake of it. A whole chapter could be written on just what happens psychologically, physically and spiritually when we really involve ourselves in being these movements. But find out for yourself. Do them and see how wonderful they are; how relaxed and fulfilled you feel afterwards.

19. *The birth position*. After the last relaxation of the previous series, put a pillow under your head, draw the knees up, feet apart, hands by the side. The feet should be about a yard apart, knees fairly high. This is the birth position used almost exclusively throughout the civilised world. One of the few

disadvantages of this posture, as against the squat, is that there is an inclination to arch the back and tense the genital and rectal area during contractions. This was why we practised the tensions and relaxing in the squat position. Therefore try to tense the abdominal muscles while keeping the lower back relaxed and genital area untensed. In a sense, as will be explained later, the process of birth is not unlike certain parts of the spontaneous movements that occur during orgasm. This may seem far-fetched when compared with the average woman's experience of birth. Nevertheless, there is some evidence to support the idea that birth should be as wild and wonderful as complete orgasm. That in most cases it is not, may simply point to the probability that most of us cannot fully surrender to spontaneous emotions and movements, and that the muscles of most women are not sufficiently well exercised or well nourished enough in the sense of present nutritional research. But it is hoped that these outlines of exercise and diet will go a long way to remedying this.

Earlier we talked about natural or instinctive postures the body assumes. It was said that because we often deny or prevent our instinctive drives we often fail to be able to assume these spontaneous postures and thus cannot experience the sense of pleasure and fulfilment arising with them. This is very true in the sex act, and also in childbirth. Virtually everyone recognises, even though they may not be very conscious of it, that during labour the contractions are spontaneous. Just as a deeper level of our being controls digestion and heartbeat, which we can interfere with or modify according to our emotions and tensions, so also this deeper instinctive, or bio-energetic level, causes contractions and the process of birth. If our habits of tension or emotional reaction interfere with the natural development of such processes, pain and dissatisfaction can occur.

Thanks to the amazing work of Wilhelm Reich as expressed in his book *The Function of the Orgasm*, it is easy to see how much habits interfere with instinctive drives, which subsequently become painful instead of blissful. For instance, in the sex act spontaneous movements cause the abdominal muscles to contract, swivelling the pelvis forward and upwards. In the man this causes deeper penetration; in the woman, a relaxation and 'giving' of the genitals. When lying on the floor, this movement causes a rising of the hips, *but not of the lumbar region*. In fact the hollow in the small of the back disappears, bringing that part of the back flat on to the floor. Also the head drops back and the mouth usually opens. When habits of emotional tension interfere with this spontaneous movement, it often happens that due to unconscious fear of genital *pleasure*, the hips draw *back* instead of swivelling up. This makes the hollow in the back more pronounced. Or else genital tension causes the body to arch stiffly up causing the lower back to lift off the floor. Such tensions, which do not allow the genital pleasure to develop into the bliss of orgasm, instead cause such feelings to be experienced as disgusting, frightening, hateful, repugnant, or painful.

We can learn an enormous amount from this in regard to childbirth. In a similar way, unconscious fears or tension can cause either a *drawing back* of the genitals during contractions, or an arching of the body upwards. The instinctive ecstasy of childbirth is also in the same way stopped from developing.

Of course, it is all very well talking about this, but is there anything we can do that will be of practical help? Well, we can watch our sexual intercourse to see whether we allow the spontaneous movements to possess us without fear. If we observe the tensions that result in pulling back the hips or arching the back, we can attempt to relax them and face the fears that underly them. For if the tension is caused by a feeling of guilt, sin, and dirtiness in regard to intercourse, then we will certainly have to face these feelings in relaxing the tension. You can also practise the movement *and feeling* of sexual 'giving' and surrender in this posture.

The following advice may cause shock in some quarters; it is nevertheless time that people know the details of this method based on modern psychology and ancient yoga. If some people doubt that such methods have ever been a part of yoga, I would agree that in this form, probably not. But any study of Tantric yoga, its principles and practices, will assure the reader that the method is developed from yoga principles, where the study of sexual relationship as an inner and outer fact is used. It is a bad reflection on our society that I should even feel the need to apologise, for the following are but natural expressions of our feelings.

In this technique, use your imagination freely. Hold in mind what has already been said about the spontaneous posture. Now imagine your response to intercourse. Allow your imagination to express itself in movement, letting the hips curve up, the head drop back quite loose and free to move, and the breath come in quick panting. Let all tension in the genitals drop away and the feeling of delight arising in the genitals develop. The aim is to let genital pleasure happen so that it relaxes all but the abdominal contraction that pulls the hips up. We also aim to become very conscious of the emotional and physical feeling of genital 'giving' and sexual surrender, or surrender to sexual feelings without sense of sin, guilt, or tension.

When this is achieved, allow any spontaneous movements of the hips to continue, although at first this may be jerky. Now realise that the contractions in this case are not to give your love and being more deeply to your partner, *but to give your love and being to the world in the form of your baby.* Nevertheless, the movement is the same, and if successful, the joy is the same also. Please realise that you are practising this movement and giving so that at childbirth it will be habitual. That is, the hips up without hollowing the back; the genitals relaxed, surrendered to spontaneous movement.

20. *Toning-up movements.* While the above ways of 'Being Movement' are quite different from the 'yoga postures' we usually read about, such postures are only a tiny part of yoga methods. Such ways of exercising as I have given have been used for centuries, but are little known. Likewise, there are some consciously motivated movements also used by various yogis, which are a great help in toning up our body. These are

very simple, but have quite a profound influence on the body. When you first use them, do so very gently and for only about thirty seconds. But as you become accustomed to them, gradually lengthen the time of practice to five or even ten minutes. At first they may cause great discomfort inside the body because they massage the internal organs. This is why you must do them gently and only for a short period. If you patiently persist, however, these discomforts will gradually disappear, and sometimes even illnesses are cured.

The first of these movements is done by standing with feet slightly apart, body relaxed, knees free to move, and not stiff. Then slowly start circling the shoulders forward, up to the ears and back and down. Let the head move as it wishes. When you are doing this easily, slightly bend the knees and let the bottom jut back a little. Do this very slowly at first to get the feel of the movement. Now begin to straighten the knees and bring the hips forward and up. In other words, in time with the shoulder circling, let a wavelike movement occur with the hips. Eventually the hips are going backwards and forwards as the knees are bending and straightening.

The next movement is very simple, yet again it has profound results. Stand upright and relaxed. Very slowly begin to circle the hips in a clockwise direction. The feet need to be apart to help balance, and at first the head stays more or less in one place, just the hips circling sideways right, backwards, left and forwards. As you get the feel of it, let the circling become wider and wider, even bending slightly forward and back as the hips swing round. In the first movement the hips were going backwards and forwards. In this one they are going round and round. After circling clockwise, then circle anti-clockwise.

The last of these movements takes a bit more energy, but is again very simple. Stand with feet apart and bend the knees slightly, taking up a position skiers or skaters take – trunk forward, bottom back. Then begin to move the hips from side to side while remaining in the position. At first keep the trunk and arms still until you get used to the movement; then move your arms as if running or skating in time with the hip movements, but do not move the feet. So in fact it is like skating standing still.

Considering that it is advisable to also practise daily relaxation and breathing, the above complete exercises may need too much time. It is therefore suggested that through personal experiment you work out a routine for yourself which fits your timetable and abilities. I would suggest rather than cut out any of the postures or exercises, they should be practised a few on one day, a few another, until you have done them all, and then start again. Or at least, incorporate all the series over a period of several sessions. But if you have the energy and the time, practise them all daily. Always rest for some minutes after the postures.

Another point is that although the routine is directly designed for the already pregnant, it is nevertheless important to realise that whenever possible parenthood should be taken very seriously, seriously enough to prepare before conception in as many ways as possible. Endeavouring to get one's body in tiptop condition is basic to all such preparation. Osteopathic adjustment to the spine; attempts to cure any digestive problems as indicated by acidity, coated tongue, etc.; treatment of any anaemia or weakness; and general all-round fitness; these should all be part of any such regime. This may sound like too much to ask. But frankly, the more you put into parenthood, the more you will get out of it. Certainly it will be more of a personally creative event.

2.

Influencing the Unborn Child

In 1962 most authorities did not believe that the unborn child could be influenced by the activities of the mother. In that year a shocked world witnessed the birth of growing numbers of malformed thalidomide babies. Yet for generations, those who had listened to their intuition had warned the public time and again that a tragedy could occur if they were not more careful in their use of medical drugs and diet. The world is still being warned that drug use during pregnancy is only part of the problem. In a world rushing headlong into the ever greater use of manufactured, synthetic and preserved foods, any number of further catastrophes still promise to mature.

Prior to 1962, it was generally believed that the placenta acted as a barrier to harmful substances ingested by the mother, or circulating in her blood. To damage a baby without killing the mother too was thought impossible. To quote from a recent scientific statement, however, 'We now know that nothing could be further from the truth. There are a number of substances which can damage a baby profoundly, particularly during the early weeks of pregnancy, probably even before the mother knows she is pregnant.' The harmful influences are listed as radiation, chemicals, notably drugs, and some infections. There is as yet no detailed knowledge of exactly what changes most drugs, such as aspirin, codein, and the host of other medical chemicals, cause in the unborn child. But in animal experiments it has been found *that almost any drug can damage the foetus*.

Dr Guttmacher, in his book, *Pregnancy and Birth*, gives possible causes of damage as: German measles during early pregnancy; the transfusion of Rh positive blood to Rh negative girls or women; excessive insulin during pregnancy for the diabetic mother; poor standard of physical, nutritive or reproductive health in the parents at conception, and in the mother during pregnancy; X-ray during pregnancy, especially to the pelvic region; general anaesthesia in pregnancy during dental and surgical procedures; air travel in unpressurised cabins before the twelfth week; children born to aged parents; medical and social drugs (smoking and alcohol, for instance).

Obviously, such statements need some comments in balancing our understanding. Despite the fact that the unborn baby can be hurt by so many factors – *virtually all of them due to the unnatural things men and women subject their bodies to*– the foetus is, nevertheless, fantastically resourceful in meeting difficulties, especially in healthy parents. This naturally applies to elderly parents also.

Quoting once more from a reasonably conservative authority, we find the statement that,

Only in recent years have we come to recognise the importance of foetal life. Its quality has a profound effect on everything that happens later to the individual. The growth and health of the foetus is influenced to some extent by its own inherited make-up, but this is profoundly influenced and modified by its environment, probably from the very moment of conception. . . . The uterus itself must be a suitable bed and container for the baby. . . . It can only do this if the mother herself is in good health, and, ideally, the mother should be free from disease and extremely well nourished throughout her pregnancy. In general, the better the health and nutrition of the mother the better will be the baby's chances of a healthy nine months in the womb and a robust delivery and survival.

Why drugs can be harmful
Having said this much, let us look in greater detail at the statements already made. For instance, why can drugs and unnatural procedures harm the unborn baby? What is meant

by 'a poor standard of physical, nutritive and reproductive health'? And what is a chemical?

As yet, very little is known as to exactly why drugs and some unnatural procedures cause the results they do. Perhaps we can gain a little insight by understanding what drugs do, and why we take them, or at least why they are used.

There are many types of drugs. Some are derived from plants or trees, such as opium, quinine, and digitalis. Although found in plants they are nearly always simply one part of the plant's chemical compound, which is extracted and concentrated. Other drugs are chemicals that are produced almost entirely artificially, either through the refining processes as in oil derivatives, or through other chemical procedures. Now drugs have entered yet another area, that of the antibiotic type, which are not inert chemicals but living moulds, as with penicillin. One can state fairly confidently that all drugs are used either to produce changes in the body, or to stop changes taking place. These are *the* reasons for drug use.

It seems that these are also *the* reasons why they are dangerous, especially during pregnancy. We need little imagination or understanding of natural processes to see why. Anything, whether plant or human, that is full grown, is difficult to alter in size, build, and basic characteristics. But the further back we go in the process of growth, the greater ability we have to direct and influence the development that will follow. In pregnancy as a whole, and in the first three months in particular, the most fantastic, even miraculous, changes are taking place. Apart from anything else, the sperm and ovum increase their weight millions of times. During these very intricate and delicate changes, any chemical or drug, which after all is specifically designed to either induce change or interfere with it, can influence the development radically.

The medical practice uses drugs because they influence the body's nervous system, functions, cells, etc., in major ways. As adults, or established children, we can sometimes survive such drugs without too violent side-effects, because our body and its processes have reached a point of stasis that protects it. The foetus has not by any means reached this stability; its whole life is fantastic change and growth.

We have seen that drugs are either synthetic substances, or chemicals taken from plants and concentrated in order to have more profound or 'concentrated' results. But the statements made by doctors say that drugs and chemicals may injure the unborn baby. Therefore, what is the difference between a drug and a chemical? Basically, most drugs are chemical substances that are used for medicinal purposes. Whereas a chemical, as the word is used above, is a chemical substance (i.e. a substance artificially produced) used for non-medical purposes. The word therefore covers a variety of chemicals used, for instance, in agriculture as fertilisers and pesticides; in the home as pesticides, food additives, flavourings, sweeteners to food and drink; as fumes, gases, water additives, etc.

Many chemicals are therefore taken into our body in the air we breathe, fluids we drink, foods we eat, and household appliances we use. At first sight these do not appear as dangerous as the use of drugs during pregnancy. It is certainly true that most of them produce nothing like the changes of, for instance, thalidomide. But at the beginning of this chapter I said that the intuitive are still warning us of coming catastrophes. It is in this area they feel one of the greatest dangers lies. This is because of several fairly logical reasons. Most of these chemicals are taken quite unconsciously. They are taken in very large amounts. Neither is there a feeling of reserve about them as with the use of drugs.

To take but two of the most commonly used chemicals, we have white sugar and white flour. Many people will feel shocked that I have named these as chemicals, yet neither of them occur naturally. Both are produced by complex procedures. Both are concentrated extracts of plants. Both produce marked changes in the body, and so could almost be called drugs. Certainly both are dangerous influences on the unborn, and the born. Why?

Some years ago, a dental expert, Dr Price, became interested in the causes of tooth decay, and also dental malformations – that is, misplaced, cramped teeth, and narrow mouth. He began to investigate, and during many years' research gradually uncovered far more than he had ever expected, or even looked for. He found that the causes were due to our change of diet, particularly white flour and white sugar. This may seem an interesting little snippet of information, one to be smiled over and forgotten, until we pause one moment in thought. Remember, I did not just say dental decay; I also said dental and mouth malformation.

Is it not a sobering thought to realise that more and more of our race, through its growing diet of chemicals, are being born with malformations? Joan Grant, during an archaeological dig in the Middle East, collected forty sets of teeth. She says that there were 'children's teeth, middle-aged teeth, teeth of men who were so old that the surface of the molars was ground almost smooth – and in none of the forty sets I collected was there a single decayed tooth, nor a jaw abscess, nor a wisdom tooth that had not grown in exact alignment with the rest.'

Please do not think that I feel white flour, white sugar, and the other chemicals we absorb are simply causing malformations in increasing numbers of unborn babies. No, it is even worse than that. What is happening is that the drugs and chemicals are doing exactly the job they were designed for – namely, producing changes in *our* body. In particular, one of the most sensitive parts of our body, the genes in our sperm and ova.

During the 1930s, Sir Robert McCarrison, a world-famous nutritionist and scientist, carried out an experiment in diet using rats. He fed groups of rats diets common among a variety of different races. The diseases suffered in each race were startlingly reproduced among the rats. But possibly an even more important experiment, in considering the results of refined and synthetic foods, was that done by Bernasek in Prague. One group of rats was fed on wheat grain, dried lucerne, margarine, cod liver oil, dried full milk, casein, calcium carbonate and salt. The other group was fed on a diet where all natural fats had been replaced by margarine with all known vitamins, minerals and trace elements added synthetically. Thus this diet was the chemical equivalent of the natural one. All of these rats, from an original 120, in four generations had died out entirely. Quoting from an article by Michael Allaby in *Here's Health*, he describes the fourth generation as follows:

From the two females remaining, two litters were produced; one litter of two young, the other of five. These seven new-born rats formed the fourth generation. Three of them died straight after birth and the other four died between the sixteenth and twenty-second days, though at first they seemed to develop normally. So, by the fourth generation the experiment came to an end – the subjects were all dead.

   From the autopsies performed on all the dead rats it was learned that the females which had appeared to be sterile had, in fact, conceived, but had reabsorbed their foetuses. The young who died all suffered from disorders arising from inadequate development of myelin, the fatty substance, containing protein, which forms a sheath to the larger nerve fibres, together with degenerative changes in the nerve cells themselves.

Considering the huge influx of processed and synthetic food-stuffs, this would suggest increasing sterility in humans, and growing abnormalities at birth.

Nutrition and health
This brings us to another of the medical statements, that a poor standard of physical, nutritive or reproductive health may contribute towards malformations. All that we do, all that we are, and how we live, influences our genes, and thus contributes towards the characteristics we pass on to our children. As may be seen later in this book, the genes are not the be-all and end-all of the child's possibilities. They may be best likened to the building material which the developing baby uses. Present scientific attitude may prefer to think of them as the master plan that controls the whole development. As we have already seen, however, thalidomide can throw

even the best genes to the devil. There are also other factors. Nevertheless, it depends very much upon the mothers of this era as to how our race develops in the next few generations.

It has always been recognised by animal breeders that the quality of the offspring is mostly due to the quality of the parents. It is important that the parents be in top form when they mate, as this too has a great influence on offspring. It has for long amazed me that people will go to such lengths and effort to bring their animals to top condition, regulate their diet carefully, see they are exercised, happy and content, to produce beautiful offspring, yet they themselves couldn't give a damn when producing offspring. They rest inadequately, eat rubbish they would never feed to their animals, mate even in the middle of an illness, and generally act as if they had not a degree of intelligence. The same people walk about saying, 'Isn't it terrible the number of babies born with cancer now.'

It is the opinion of many nutritionists that most, if not all, cases of children born dead, sick, malformed, or who die shortly after birth, could be avoided by correct diet and living. In America today, the most 'civilised' and therefore the most badly fed country due to enormous food refinement, it is estimated that one in six men cannot father a child, 1 in 200 babies is born deformed, 600,000 have cerebral palsy, and 1 out of 100 babies is mentally retarded.

The adults are in an even worse state as their impoverished diet leads to further degeneration of health. One in ten is likely to become a patient of a mental hospital. Sixteen million have heart defects. Nearly a million are being treated for cancer. There are eight million arthritics, and three million diabetics. Also multiple sclerosis adds another 250,000; muscular dystrophy 200,000, and T.B. another 400,000. Obviously, the unnamed sicknesses would take the total into fear-raising numbers. If you believe that this is the fate of mankind, to suffer and die, then it reflects the sickness of mind our society lives in. Investigations carried out by Sir Robert McCarrison, on the Hunzas of the Himalayas, showed a race to shame our 'civilised' races. There were no kidney diseases, no cancer, no heart conditions, no ulcers, tooth decay, digestive illnesses, arthritis, malformations, or other illnesses. Neither were there any criminals, mental illness, homosexuality, alcoholism, drug addiction, delinquency, or social disturbances. They live to a great old age with all faculties, and death is usually quick and painless; a laying aside of the body. Adelle Davis, in her book *Let's Eat Right to Keep Fit*, also mentions the researches of Dr Price as reported in his book *Nutrition and Physical Degeneration*.

He tells of a people with erect postures, unbelievable endurance, and cheerful even dispositions. These people had excellent bone structure; their faces and jaws were so wide and well developed that their teeth were not crowded together, and stayed free from decay just as their bodies stayed free from disease. The statistics concerning the incidence of cancer, ulcers, high blood pressure, tuberculosis, heart and kidney diseases, muscular dystrophy, multiple sclerosis, and cerebral palsy were zero, zero, zero in every case. Names for these diseases were unknown and unneeded. Dr Price found no physicians, surgeons, psychiatrists, no crime, no prisons, no mental illness and no institutions for the insane, feeble-minded, alcoholics, drug addicts; no child delinquency, no homosexuality. Every mother nursed her babies; a nonfunctional breast was unheard of. Mental, moral and emotional health accompanied physical health.

Many other studies of so-called 'primitives' revealed groups in Africa, South America, and elsewhere, having the same health and well-being. These investigations, in similar studies of such communities who had been influenced by the 'civilised' races, even though living in the same area, but now eating civilised foods such as white sugar and white flour, found tooth decay, faulty bone structures, crime, sexual immorality, perversions, ulcers, colitis, and so on through the list of civilised sickness.

Medical and social research have also uncovered a mass of information the public knows little or nothing about. A few snippets of such information that refer to pregnancy, childlessness, and malformations are as follows.

Studies have shown that smoking not only results in a

smaller baby, but in some cases in infertility. Males have shown dead sperm due to smoking. Tests on rats given nicotine resulted in decreased fertility. A German study revealed its influence on sexual hormones generally, resulting in greater incidence of sterility, frigidity, miscarriage and menstrual disturbance amongst smokers. Animals absorbing the equivalent of twenty cigarettes daily had a ten times higher rate of still-births than usual.

The Lancet and *British Medical Journal* both draw notice to the fact that cortisone taken during pregnancy can cause cleft palate in the baby. Other factors have also been found to cause the same results. Vitamin A and the B vitamins, especially B_6, when withheld in animal diets, caused harelip in progeny. Experimenters could cause this at will simply by withholding these nutrients. Similar results have been noted in humans.

Dr Kugelman states that the increase in mental backwardness or illness in the newborn is often due to insufficient nutrition in pregnancy. The results of a seven-year test were given in the 1955 March issue of *Time*. 2,400 women took part in the test. They were from working-class families with poor diets. Some were given pills of no nutritional value. The others received nutritional supplements during their pregnancies. It was shown that the children from those women on supplemental nutrition were indeed of higher intelligence generally than those on the placebo.

A fascinating story is told by Dr Anna Szasz of Budapest. She has worked for many years on the treatment of mongoloid children, and has discovered that vitamin E supplement given from birth causes gradual but very definite positive development to take place. One of her patients, a woman of middle age, gave birth to three mongoloid children, each one worse than the last. She then became pregnant again, but this time Dr Szasz put her on a high protein diet with plenty of vegetables and liver. She was also given full vitamin supplementation with an emphasis on vitamin E. Her baby was born at the right time, perfectly sound and healthy.

Still on the subject of mongolism, Dr Rapaport researched

into the incidence of mongol births in areas with fluoridated water supplies. He found that in areas with only up to 0.2 mlg of fluorine per litre of water, 34.15 mongols per 100,000 births occurred. But in areas where the fluorine level was 1.0 to 2.6 mlg per litre, 71.59 mongols were born per 100,000 births.

As pointed out elsewhere, Dr Carlton Fredericks (Ph.D.) reports that still-births rose 150 per cent in areas that became fluoridated. And animal research has shown fluoride dissolves forming heart tissue in embryos.

Experiments have shown that animals eating only proteins that have been cooked die out by the fourth generation. Considering how little uncooked foods people now eat, this naturally suggests a threat to correct reproduction. The animals developed malfunction increasingly in each genera-tion. The same is happening to thousands of people in our society now. Our very babies, fed on a 'formula' instead of at their mothers' breasts, are literally initiated into the death-dealing process at birth. Because the difficulties do not show immediately is no sign that the changes are not occurring in the baby's body. If the baby has to have a formula prepara-tion, the threat can be offset by feeding living protein as soon as possible. Pasteurised milk, killed as it is by heat, is not among the living protein class.

During the years 1924–29, 20,061 babies were investigated at the Chicago Infant Welfare Centre. To quote from Alan Moyle's book *About Nature Cure*, the facts arising from this investigation showed the enormous difference in death rates between breast-fed and bottle-fed babies.

	Infants	Deaths	Percentage
Entirely breast-fed	9,794	15	0.15
Partially breast-fed	8,605	59	0.7
Artificially fed	1,707	144	8.4

Reaching a high standard of health
Having looked at some of the negative aspects of how the un-born baby can be influenced, we may turn our attention to more constructive features. If we consider what can cause

detrimental results, we can begin to see clearly what will cause beneficial results. To summarise, we said that virtually all artificial and unnatural influences can cause injury to the development. This is because, being unnatural, the mother's and the baby's body have to attempt an adjustment to it, or normal functions are interfered with. This applies to all drugs and those chemicals which induce harmful changes, including such as 'the pill', and those taken as food. The prospective parents, and the pregnant mother especially, should attempt to reach a high standard of health, on a whole-food, and as far as possible raw-food, diet. This will be explained in greater detail in the chapter on diet. All influences that interfere with natural processes should be avoided. Great attention should be given to the body's needs, such as sufficient exercise, rest, social relaxation, breathing, toilet, self-expression and reception of love and affection, and so on. Undoubtedly, with many of us, it will be the loving and disciplined work of several generations attempting to live in the right way, before the bodies produced are the completely beautiful and radiantly healthy temples of the soul they should be.

There is then the other side to influencing the unborn child that is at present still smiled upon as superstition by most doctors and scientists. This is the influence upon how it will look, and specifically upon the nature of its personality. Obviously, nearly all that is written about this subject has been by those I have called the intuitive section of society. Just as these were the first to point out the physical dangers of pre-natal influence, they are also the first to point out the possibilities of psychological influence. So far, it is only the physical influence that science can see for itself. Also, much rubbish has been said and written in the name of the intuitives concerning this subject. Nevertheless, there does seem to be some very serious evidence and statements worthy of consideration. To understand these statements, we have to understand how the intuitive mind works. It does not reach its conclusions by reasoning from revealed 'facts'. It appears, in its highest form, to directly experience things, or perceive directly without the use of intellect. The difficulty then lies in attempting to express what has been experienced. It is as difficult as a scientist attempting to explain to a layman the complex relationships of biochemic activity. Fortunately, many of these intuitive realisations are to a small extent now observed scientifically.

For instance, one of the intuitive statements is that the unborn baby has, from the start, an aware relationship with the mother. This is where we begin to have difficulty in explaining intuitive terms, simply because such issues are not common knowledge. But by 'awareness' is *not* meant thought. Nevertheless, the baby is *not* a dead thing. All living things have awareness in some degree, and the unborn baby is certainly not a piece of rock, but has a high level of awareness. Just as a bad relationship with the mother can cause psychological difficulties in the child, and later the adult, simply because the adult develops from the child, so can problems experienced by the unborn baby cause difficulties in the child. I have noticed in one of my own sons that from the earliest part of his life, in fact from birth, he has been far more cautious and in need of security than my other children. From the time he could speak he would never allow a fire to be left on in his room; he did not walk until three due to fear of falling. Babies are often born with psychological problems. In the case of my son, this is possibly due to the difficulty of his breech birth, and its shock and strain. In others, there is evidence to show that it has preceded birth.

Meanwhile, taking it as an unproven possibility, what can we do about it? The whole force about much that has been said in regard to pre-natal influence is its inference that one can 'put it on' like a regime for slimming. This influence, from the scanty information at hand so far, is not a thing we can switch on or off. It lies in the whole realm of how the woman reacts to the fact there is another being developing within her. It lies in whether she feels resentment, fear, fulfilment, love, guilt, desire to abort, and the infinity of other human feelings. Is the baby wanted? Why is it wanted, or not wanted? Is the relationship with the coming baby a mature, problem-facing one? Some have a baby as one might have a doll, others in an attempt to cement a marriage, or through family or social pressure. All these attitudes constitute a form of relationship with the unborn, and of course the born, baby, and have tremendous influence upon it. Any pressing psychological problems we may have, such as frigidity, feelings of uncleanness in regard to sex, great insecurity, deep depressions, and so on, also constitute a relationship that influences the baby, even prior to birth. Ideally, one should attempt to resolve such problems prior to pregnancy. As nobody is perfect however, we cannot, and indeed it is unrealistic and itself a problem to aim at human perfection. What we can aim at is the admittance of our weaknesses and problems, and the attempt to recognise them as difficult areas that should not control the important decisions in our life. What we can do is to see our life as a field of amazing possibilities that can be worked on, gradually moulded and released. What we can do is to attempt self-understanding, and through it growth to greater maturity and self-expression.

Let us face facts. What influences the baby most, whether born or unborn, is the whole structure of the mother and father's personality, and all the actions and interactions that arise from this. It is unrealistic to think we can suddenly change this pattern of our moods, fears, preferences, hates and morals, just because a baby is planned or on its way. But it is not unrealistic, either before or during pregnancy, to look upon oneself as a problem that can be gradually worked on and understood. We therefore have to admit that one of the greatest factors in influencing our children is what we have already done with our life. How much ability, patience, understanding, perseverance, gentleness, lovingness, co-operation, and insight we have cultivated. History proves it as at least a general fact that an Abraham Lincoln is not born from the womb of a hateful, vengeful woman. It is also now recognised that any long discipline of mind, emotion or body can alter our genetic make-up. In his book *Raja Yoga*, Yesudian, talking on this subject, gives the example of Nijinsky, the great ballet dancer. For several generations his family had been dancers; now, the very bone structure of his foot had altered from the normal, enabling him to leap quite extraordinarily.

Special efforts during pregnancy, whether of diet, exercise, or mind, do seem to count for a lot, however. Obviously one does not have to be a great musician to give birth to a musical prodigy, or a great runner to give birth to an athlete. It helps if it is 'in the family', but it is by no means necessary. Again, it is the relationships between parents and child that count for most; the depth, discipline, sincerity, encouragement, example of love, that help or hinder the expression of what the child is. We do not create the child, but as parents we do hand over much in the way of physique and health, attitudes, understanding, that are the building materials, the foundation of the child's future life as an independent being. The special discipline during pregnancy can play a very real part in this. One could, of course, quote cases like that of Amy Johnson's mother who, during pregnancy, thought of little else except aeroplanes and flying. But such cases are unusual. What can be done is to attempt to live in as great a harmony with ourself as possible. That is, attempt to supply what our body needs in the way of nutrition, exercise and rest. Also we can indulge in our special interests, or those things that bring great pleasure and happiness. Read again the books that have moved you, or opened depths of realisation and feeling. Listen to the music you love. Rest often. Indulge your desire to talk or cuddle or swim, or whatever it is that brings lasting fulfilment and a sense of well-being. Avoid stress as much as possible. But not in the negative sense of avoiding challenges, problems, or running away from difficulties which, if only you faced up to them, would begin to be resolved. In other words, as much as possible be yourself, your real self, the self you have always longed to be deep down, but which fears and pressures have prevented you from realising. This is all your baby requires of you. Undoubtedly though, the offering of self to Life, or God, as a channel for the expression of Life's hidden splendour, has more influence in creating a beautiful baby than any other single factor.

Gayelord Hauser tells us, in his book *The New Diet Does It*, of an interesting approach to this question. He says:*

Once when I was in Paris, I stood in a museum admiring 'The Thinker' by Rodin. Beside me was a young American woman, an acquaintance, attractive enough by ordinary standards. On close scrutiny, however, her face showed lines of dissatisfaction and unhappiness. She had told me her story; how the children had been ill all winter; there had been a siege of pneumonia besides continuous colds; and a small son had been operated on for mastoid. The winter had left her so fatigued from worry and sleepless nights and hard physical work that her husband had insisted on the holiday in Paris and had arranged for his mother to stay with the children.

Such stories are common enough, but invariably sad to anyone who holds the conviction that these illnesses are needless and can be prevented.

'How I wish I might be an artist,' she exclaimed wistfully. 'It must be wonderful to be able to create such beauty for others to see. I spend my life cooking, shopping and nursing the children. I'm nothing, really, just a *Hausfrau*. It makes one seem so useless.'

She had touched on one of my deepest convictions: that every mother can be an artist, a sculptor, that she has it in her power to create and help develop live, vital beings.

'Don't you see that you can create beauty in building beautiful children?' I asked her. 'Rodin first worked in clay, then in bronze; you work with living flesh. Just as he moulded his works of art, so you are moulding the bodies and spirits of your children. Just as he spent hours in shaping and reshaping clay, you spend hours in shopping and cooking. When the cooking is done with care, and foods which build health are purchased, when those foods are prepared to save their vital elements to build beauty, then the kitchen has dignity as great as the studio of any famous artist.'

Gradually I could see her wistfulness and dissatisfaction disappear; her attitude toward housework and child care changed.

Years later when I met her at a lecture I was giving in Philadelphia she showed me three wonderful, glowing children. She had created three works of art which were beautiful not only in body, but in mind and spirit.

* Extract from *The New Diet Does It* reprinted by permission of Faber and Faber Ltd.

3.

Feeding the Unborn Child

The unborn baby is often described as a perfect parasite. By this physiologists mean that the baby takes from the mother all the nutritive factors it needs, even if this is to the detriment of the mother. Some women lose teeth during pregnancy due to the baby's need for calcium, and the drain on the mother's calcium supply. Similarly, the expectant mother may easily become anaemic unless her absorption of iron from food equates that taken from her by the baby. The amount of vitamin C can also be very much higher in the foetus than in the mother, showing its need of this vitamin.

At first sight this may lead us to believe that dietary disciplines are needed solely for the mother in order to prevent *her* deficiencies. If the mother is not including certain minerals and vitamins in her diet, however, the baby will not be able to obtain enough from her blood supply anyway. The attitude on the part of many medical practitioners not to be concerned by what the pregnant mother is eating, seems, from their own evidence, to be terribly shortsighted. As Dr Guttmacher has said, many childless couples can produce healthy children when their own level of health is improved. It must be obvious to any thinking person that if the health of the womb and developing placenta are not adequate, not only can this lead to childlessness, and miscarriage, but also to inadequate functioning for the surviving child. A personal feeling is that many of the congenital conditions that some babies arrive with, could have been prevented by a deeper interest in radiant health for the mother. I am sure some congenital illnesses will be traced to this source. Quite apart from this, the course of the woman's pregnancy can be different if common-sense measures are followed, and the birth itself short, pleasant, and without complications. There is certainly no need whatsoever for so many women to suffer from varicose veins, constipation, piles, anaemia, exhaustion, septicaemia, loss of figure after birth, and the host of other problems often accepted as a 'natural' part of pregnancy. Not only this, the very nature and body of our child can be more beautiful if we work *with* nature in its creative processes, instead of hindering and obstructing it. Therefore we will look at the details of diet, and how we can apply them. As stated already, it is better to start long before pregnancy, but it is never too late.

Health questionnaire

Let us begin by checking our health as thoroughly as we can. The following questions will help you to see in greater detail just what you may need to improve the general standard of your health. A list of vitamin-rich foods is given later.

Hair

Is your hair dry, falling, scurfy, or with broken ends? Is it losing its colour already? Pet owners can always tell the health of their animal from the condition of its hair. Yet people hardly ever take an honest look at their own hair as an indication of general health. I know from experience that dry and rapidly falling hair, with scurf, is a sign of poor nutrition. Gayelord Hauser points out that the Chinese race have very little baldness, and suggests this is due to their diet, rich in B vitamins. Similarly, the rural Irish enjoy beautiful hair, and often their diet includes much Irish moss and iodine. If your hair is in bad condition, then a diet rich in B vitamins and vitamin A is indicated. Also natural yogurt, black treacle and kelp tablets or powder help, as do raw fruit and vegetables, as the silica in the skin is used to build hair cells. For a very quick change in hair condition, a diet which includes plenty of raw fruit and vegetables, with a vitamin A supplement and brewer's yeast, will bring results. (Halibut oil capsules and brewer's yeast powder.)

Eyes

Many eye conditions can be either helped, or cured, by fulfilling the body's needs. Sore eyes, sandiness, night-blindness, forming cataracts, or eyes too sensitive to light, suggest the need for larger amount of vitamins A, B and C.

Nose and throat

Do you suffer from catarrh, sinusitis, tonsillitis, sore throat? These frequently show a body loaded with poisons and toxins and undernourished in the enzymes, vitamins and minerals found in raw foods. The cleansing diet, outlined later, is indicated, followed by a diet rich in vitamins A and C.

Teeth and gums

As shown in the first chapter, one of the curses of our civilised diet is unhealthy teeth. Not only is this due to the chewing of soft foods and chemical sugar, but also highly concentrated starches as in white flour; and lack of raw foods. It is also due to deficiencies of the necessary minerals and vitamins. Bleeding gums and mouth sores are another sign of nutritional insufficiencies. In experiments where laboratory animals were given insufficient vitamin C, a condition similar to pyorrhoea was produced. But any person who suffers pyorrhoea can prove to themselves that this is a sign of deficiency in vitamin C and the B vitamins by taking 500 mlg of vitamin C daily for a while, along with a B supplement, and increasing the oranges and green leaves eaten. The pyorrhoea will promptly disappear.

Do you have any dead or infected teeth? If so, have these seen to at all costs, as they are often the foci for innumerable ills. Adequate vitamin C, D and A are necessary for healthy, pain-free teeth, along with phosphorus, calcium and the B vitamins.

Chest

Do you suffer from bronchial infections? Is your breathing deep and regular? Do you suffer from allergies, or asthma? All can be helped or cured through correct nutrition as long as the other aspects of life are also watched and cared for. Allergies can be helped or healed by regular large doses of vitamin C (100 mlg each meal), or in severe attacks, 100 mlg every two hours. While vitamin A in large amounts can prevent or cure sinus trouble, hay fever and bronchial troubles, A and C should be taken together in these cases. Asthma sometimes responds to adequate supplies of calcium in diet and in tablet form. During an attack, Gayelord Hauser recommends two or three calcium tablets every hour, and the use of 100 mlg of vitamin E after each meal. This aids the oxygenation of tissues. Other helpful and sometimes curative remedies are to lay thin slices of onion on a plate and spread honey over them; cover, and leave for eight hours, then take a teaspoonful of the resulting syrup four times a day. It is wise to practise the yoga breathing methods also. Learn the abdominal breathing as described later, and practise very slow breathing in this way, each day. The cleansing diet should be used to clear catarrh if it exists. The recommended vitamins should wherever possible be taken in foods or juices rather than tablets.

Muscles

Is there a tendency to cramps, muscular ache, weakness, etc? There is definite information from research to show that a lack of calcium, vitamins D and B, and magnesium causes cramps. Lack of magnesium also contributes to muscular weakness, and convulsions. As this is easily taken as Epsom salt, it is a simple matter to right. Naturally, healthy muscles need adequate protein intake, and can be strengthened by large amounts of vitamin E in the daily diet, along with frequent exercise. Even severe muscular illnesses, such as sclerosis, can sometimes be cured by sufficient vitamin E.

Stomach

Is there acidity, indigestion, inability to digest foods? Nowadays, with the increasing use of antibiotics taken orally, many people cannot properly digest their food due to the antibiotics having destroyed the necessary bacteria and enzymes in the intestines. This can be usually put right by stopping the antibiotics, and eating raw foods swarming with 'germs'; or taking Florus, which contains the bacteria. Acidity is nearly always the result of eating wrong foods, lack of B vitamins, or a mixture of concentrated sugar, as in white sugar, and concentrated starch, as in white flour, which produces a tremendously acid stomach reaction when eaten together. The mixture of starches and protein in high quantities also leads to acidity. Therefore, alkaline meals should be taken, such as all fruit (uncooked, unsweetened, except with honey), which will right this.

The B vitamins, as in brewer's yeast powder, greatly aid the condition if the mentioned food mixtures are avoided as much as possible, and less concentrated starches, such as wholewheat flour, Barbados sugar, or honey, and potatoes in their jackets are used; but generally eat less starch and sugar. The apple fast is an extremely quick cure for acidity, while a couple of days on just plain, natural yogurt can be used to restore the proper bacteria balance to the digestive system.

Intestines

Do you suffer from painful flatulence, constipation, diarrhoea, piles? These disturbances show deficiencies in several ways, especially of the B vitamins and some minerals. These can be found in brewer's yeast and black treacle, both of which should be taken during pregnancy, whether you are constipated or not. This applies also to diarrhoea, which may be due to lack of magnesium and B vitamins, and when not due to an infection, shows a very unbalanced diet generally. In cases of flatulence, constipation, piles, or diarrhoea, a level teaspoon of Irish moss or agar agar, taken beaten into milk with the main meal, will greatly help or cure. Use it more frequently if necessary. It is extremely nutritious. The aim is to produce formed but very soft stools. If these do not occur, take larger doses of the Irish moss, but make sure your diet is adequate in wholewheat flour and raw foods. Many people find bananas cure constipation. If the stools become as suggested, piles, painful flatulence, and possibly the unsightly varicose veins of some pregnant women will disappear. This is because hard, withheld, stools, press on the veins up the spine, and cause blockage in circulation. In difficult cases, add half a cup of wheatgerm to the daily diet as well as the above suggestions. Again, yogurt and/or apples can be used as suggested above.

Bladder

Bed wetting can sometimes be cured by an adequate intake of magnesium, found in Epsom salt, dolomite tablets, nuts, soya beans, spinach, kale, and leafy green vegetables. Cystitis may show inadequacy of vitamin A in the diet.

Circulation and veins

If you have a poor circulation, varicose veins, blue patches or splotched skin, correct diet can often work miracles. For varicose veins the section on 'Intestines' should be carefully read, as constipation or delayed stools have a direct relationship with this unsightly condition. Once this aspect is being dealt with, high doses of vitamin E and C are likely to speed the cure enormously. 500 mlg of vitamins C and E daily will usually remove the varicosities quickly. The poor circulation is aided by the E and C, and needs the B vitamins also – niacin in particular is necessary for healthy circulation, but it is best taken as in brewer's yeast, dates, peanuts, etc.

Skin

Is your skin lacking a healthy pink, or glow if you are a dark-skinned person? Do you have boils, pimples, dryness or itching? Those who have changed from a poor diet to one rich in vitamins and minerals have noticed tremendous improvement in their skin, especially where the diet is rich in vitamins A and E. These two need each other for correct utilisation. Iron so plays a large part in skin tone due to it being the 'red' of the blood that carries the oxygen. If you are pale, definitely check your iron and vitamin intake, and if the skin is in poor condition, take extra E and A. An over-indulgence in white sugar and white flour often results in poor skin condition, and can be corrected by a more alkaline diet, and one high in protein.

Nerves

Under this heading must be lumped insomnia, nervous tension, alcoholism, headaches, and many other illnesses of 'nervous' origin. Many such conditions arise from psycho-logical disturbances that are only indirectly helped by diet. Nevertheless, even severe cases of madness, schizophrenia, confusion and depression have been cured by nutritional methods. In many cases the B-complex vitamins are badly needed, as in alcoholism, nervous tension, and some head-aches. Other times, as in migraine headaches and period pains, vitamin C, iron, magnesium, calcium and vitamin E can cure or help. Insomnia has responded time and time again to calcium and magnesium. Adelle Davis suggests putting two or three calcium tablets and a glass of milk on the bedside table just prior to retiring, to be used each hour of wakeful-ness. Calcium tablets should include vitamin D for proper assimilation, as do Gayelord Hauser's tablets. But perhaps kelp tablets are the best way of taking calcium. For those with insomnia, brewer's yeast tablets at meals, and kelp tablets suggested above, should be of more natural help than any sleeping tablet. This is especially necessary for many women during menstruation. One of the most beneficial of yoga methods for 'nerves' in general, is to practise *very* slow, deep, breathing for at least five minutes daily. The breathing must be as slow as possible without causing gasp-ing.

Anaemia

In recent years, nutritional research has made the terrific breakthrough of at last being able to quickly cure pernicious anaemia with vitamin B_{12} injections. However, general anaemia may be caused through inadequate protein, iron, taking of sulpha drugs, lack of iodine, cobalt, copper, vitamin E and the B vitamins. In other words, unbalanced diet, generally extended for many years. Foods which contain acid, such as buttermilk, yogurt, sour fruits and citrus fruits, aid the assimilation of iron or iron tablets. Vitamin C is also a necessary acid. Concentrated carbohydrates decrease assimilation, as do antacid tablets. Wheatgerm, black treacle and most green vegetables are very rich in iron. But they only become really effective in a well-balanced diet.

Although what I have said above, giving details of vitamins and minerals, makes a good diet sound very complex, the basis of yoga diet is really extremely simple. The way to find your own understanding of it is to build up a mental picture of a human being in natural surroundings, and following their own instinctive appetite. For instance, groups of children, at various schools, have been allowed to eat what they like instead of only what is put before them. Although at times this seemed to lead to extremes, like the little boy who consumed eight eggs straight off, over a period of time a balanced diet was achieved. The same thing has been done in family life, where the parents in a 'free' family have allowed their children to eat what they like when they like. The argument is that in nature there are no set meal times, and creatures are led by instinct to eat the things they need.

True, like animals, we too are expressions of life. What such writers fail to see, however, is that animals in their natural state are *only given a choice of natural, unprocessed foods*! When a 'free' family allow their children to eat what they like, they are not, as they claim, being 'natural' when the child is allowed unlimited sweets, processed foods, devitalised flour and packaged goods. The only time a 'free' family could achieve a natural diet would be by limiting the child's choice to natural, unprocessed foods. I use the 'free' family merely as an example. I am not suggesting you do the same. This might be too radical for you. But the simplicity of the yoga diet is certainly summed up in what I have just said.

You are a living being. Without the mysterious process of life you would not exist. Life in us consumes food to build a physical body; and the best foods we can offer Life are those that Life itself made – natural fruits and vegetables, cereals and seeds, unrefined and not destroyed by our human handwork.

Therefore, to summarise the simplicity of yoga diet as I am describing it, by all means eat at fixed meal times, but surround yourself only with wholesome foods, as much as possible uncooked and unrefined. To help you understand this more fully though, let us look at why raw foods are so necessary.

Cooked versus raw – pills versus food
Some types of food are definitely advantageous cooked. Meat, for instance, is too rampant with harmful bacteria, parasite eggs and toxins to be best eaten raw. For many, a food does not seem appetising unless cooked, or disguised, or covered in sauces. In general this can be accepted, and in the case of egg whites, it is actually necessary as they are poisonous uncooked. The pregnant or childless woman is in a different situation, however. Both have a need for maximum physical efficiency and health, and the pregnant woman also has a tremendous responsibility to the unborn. Because of this, it may be either necessary or beneficial to partake largely of raw foods.

Why is this? In the first place, most of us realise that heat produces changes in chemical composition. This is very noticeable in regard to milk, the whole composition of which is changed when sterilised or pasteurised. So vast a change is thus accomplished that calves fed solely on pasteurised milk die. This is because many of the nutrients in the milk are either destroyed, lost, or become incapable of proper absorption by the system. The figures already given of child deaths on bottle feeding show similar dangers. The same holds true in regard to any foodstuff that is cooked. Changes and losses occur of which we are only just beginning to be aware. Vitamin C is one of the great losses due to cooking, as it is largely destroyed by heat. As we need so much of it, such losses are not only criminal, they are downright dangerous to our well-being. Many minerals and other vitamins are similarly lost or changed. Enzymes in living plant cells are destroyed by heat. This causes harmful digestive activities to take place. Apart from this, the chlorophyll content of green leaves has a greater stimulus on red blood cell promotion than iron therapy; causes greater efficiency in respiration and nitrogen metabolism in cells; increases use of available proteins, balances blood-pressure, decreases insulin needs; aids wound healing; removes unpleasant body odours and increases circulation.

We must realise as well that the vitamins listed are simply those aspects of foods that have so far been discovered. Much, if not most, of natural food constituents in their relationship with each other, and cell structure, still remain unknown. Tests have begun to prove that all the vitamins and minerals interact in digestion and body utilisation. Most of the leading nutritionists realise that supplementary vitamins work most efficiently if used with a background of the other vitamins. As already pointed out, rats fed purely on synthetic nutrients died out in four generations. This is most assuredly due to the fact that we do not know the full constituents of natural, living foods, and thus cannot synthesise them. Another interesting experiment on plants showed that if a plant were fed purely artificial foods it could not use them efficiently for its development. When natural compost was fed to a separate root, not only did the plant thrive, but there was something in the compost that enabled it to make efficient use of the artificial fertilisers. There is possibly something in natural, raw foods, especially if compost grown, that has a similar effect on our body. Quite apart from which, clinical experience and the results gained by thousands of individuals who have turned to a greater use of raw foods, have proved that maximum health demands a daily intake of raw foods, especially green leaves. Even one meal per day devoted to this will work wonders. These women who have already had a child on an ordinary diet will see the difference for themselves in continued health throughout pregnancy, and the avoidance of swollen ankles, varicose veins, and septicaemia.

It is therefore far better to get the necessary vitamins and minerals from a wholesome diet rather than from tablets. In many cases, however, the fact that such tablets are available is invaluable, and often life saving. But in using them we must realise that too many vitamins, like too much food, become toxins that will clog the body rather than heal it. After all, part of health depends upon sufficient exercise, and if our system is not stimulated by attempting to extract its nutrition from natural foods, but is made lazy by being spoonfed with supplements, some forces may well atrophy if left for long periods. Although tablets such as kelp, brewer's yeast, and a few others, are foods not supplements. On the other hand, we may have vitamin and mineral deficiencies that have built up over *generations*, and thus need enormous doses of these nutrients. In all cases though, they should be taken against the background of a wholesome diet, which brings us to the detailed study of diet itself.

Below I will give a variety of diets to meet various needs. That is, sometimes a special diet is needed to cleanse the body, or to help remove some illness or condition. Later, various conditions will be listed, with details describing what can be done for them.

Cleansing diet
Many health clinics and naturopaths use fasting as a means of cleansing the body of accumulated poisons, toxins and wastes that have built up through years of wrong diet or overeating. As the discipline of fasting is not a thing many people can bring themselves to do, there is a quicker, possibly more effective and definitely easier way. This is the 'apple diet' recommended by Edgar Cayce. In three days it can cleanse the body completely, as well as removing much fatty tissue where necessary. It is very simple and easy, requiring one to eat nothing but apples for three days. These must be raw,

and as fresh as possible. No tea, coffee, alcohol or tobacco should be taken, as these are some of the very poisons being cleansed out. Literally nothing else should be taken. On the evening of the third day, half a cupful of olive oil should be taken before going to bed. This aids the lymphatic system to complete its cleansing. The next day should begin one of the full diets listed, but making sure not to gorge, but eat a little often for the first day. In fact, a pint of warm milk or natural yogurt with honey, and two dessertspoons of wheat-germ should be the first meal.

It is best to use this diet when one has little work to do. A Friday, Saturday and Sunday would be ideal, if one could rest on the Saturday and Sunday, or any days of least effort, but people who have a fair amount of weight on them will seldom feel tired on this diet. It is also best to avoid following it for longer than one day if already pregnant.

Another method is to cut out all starches, refined sugar and carbohydrates for one week, and eat only salads, without potatoes, or nuts, cream, etc., but only raw vegetables such as carrots, lettuce, tomatoes, celery, peppers, onions, radishes, watercress, cucumber, raw peas, cabbage; with any type of raw fruit, such as pineapple, grapes, limes, grapefruit, berries, peaches, melons – but no bananas. One pint of fat-free yogurt can also be taken daily, if necessary. This diet is of great help to sufferers of sciatica, rheumatism, catarrh, acidity, etc.

For those who suffer from severe intestinal or digestive disturbance, or illnesses similar to dysentery, diarrhoea, flatulence, indigestion, intestinal infections, food poisoning, and so on, another type of fast is extremely beneficial. This is an all-yogurt diet. For at least two days eat nothing but yogurt. It can easily be made by mixing a dessertspoon of plain, natural yogurt with each pint of milk. Beat the yogurt in, and stand the milk in a warm place such as an airing cupboard. Use whole milk for this, i.e. with cream. You will need at least four pints of yogurt each day. If there is no bowel movement, use an enema each day, and on the first day after the fast. This is a very simple diet, but very beneficial. Take no tea, coffee, or other foods or drinks during the diet. Eat yogurt every hour. That is about a cupful to half a pint or more, depending on appetite. The idea is to eat little, but often. No attempt is being made to starve, so eat what your appetite demands. Use no sugar. If you must use a sweetener, use a little honey, but not much.

These cleansing diets reduce weight, clear catarrh, skin, eyes, cleanse intestines and cure acidity, indigestion, piles, blood conditions, etc. The all raw fruit and vegetable diet can be taken while pregnant, if it is necessary to cleanse the body.

Weight-gaining diet
It must be made very clear that during pregnancy, unless you are painfully thin, it is best to either gain a little, or stay about the same weight. If you are heavy, then even weight loss during pregnancy is all right, as long as *it is done on a nutritious diet*, and not on appetite suppressors.

Gayelord Hauser gives the following as a sample of weight-gaining daily diet.

Breakfast: 8 ounces citrus juice, chopped dates and nuts with cream, ½ cup cooked wheatgerm eaten with blackstrap molasses and top of milk, 1 slice of wholemeal bread, toasted if desired. 1 glass of milk, or hot milk beverage. One vitamin and mineral supplement capsule.

(Gayelord Hauser suggests a lot of vitamin A in his diet, but I have found that it is easy to take too much. It then acts as a poison, causing headaches, nose bleeds, etc. I have therefore replaced his suggestion with a V.M. capsule.)

Mid-morning: 1 tablespoon of brewer's yeast (or equal in tablets) with fruit juice or yogurt.

Luncheon: Fruit salad, egg in some form, wholewheat bread and butter, a glass of yogurt, or yogurt with molasses.

Mid-afternoon: A very ripe banana – or apricot and prune juice – with peanuts.

Dinner: Salad, with tomatoes, carrots, nuts, raisins, liver or meat of choice, potato in jacket, milk drink, fruit compote, with wholewheat biscuit.

Supper: Brewer's yeast or tablets to equivalent of one tablespoon, fruit juice and yogurt.

This is merely a suggestion, and the *full diet* may be better for weight gain.

Weight-losing diet

Any woman who is overweight runs greater risk in childbearing than a slim or medium-weight woman. If you are pregnant, such reductions must be done under supervision of a doctor. If not pregnant, the cleansing diets are excellent for reducing. I have found however, that a fully balanced diet often causes weight reduction. Therefore, even in pregnancy, without doctor's supervision, the following full diet may be helpful.

Breakfast: First thing on rising, 2 dessertspoons of brewer's yeast powder mixed with milk and water to make a cupful, with a slice of wholewheat bread and honey. After washing, etc., i.e. about one and a half hours later, a poached egg, and cup of yogurt with dates, raisins and banana in it.

It has been discovered that our energy level during the day is enormously influenced by what we eat for breakfast. A high protein breakfast with a little fat, carbohydrate and sugar, causes a high energy level. This is particularly so if milk proteins, as in yogurt are supplied.

Midday, or mid-morning: Because a pregnant woman has less room in her stomach, it is better if she eats several small but nutritious meals a day, rather than three large ones. Once per day, a purely alkaline meal should be taken, and this meal is often the most opportune. Therefore, depending on appetite or taste: one pear, and two oranges *or* raw carrot, dried fruit and apple, *or* three to four apples, or slices of pineapple. The principle is to have a small meal consisting only of alkaline, uncooked foods. (See section on acid and alkaline foods.) If you have a midday meal, change these meals round to suit your timetables.

Mid-afternoon: 2 dessertspoons of wheatgerm. Place in a cup and half fill with water, then top up with yogurt or milk. Slice of bread, figs or dates.

Evening meal: Salad, consisting of something like tomato, celery, raisins, peanuts or any nuts, any chopped dried fruit, lettuce (green leaves), raw carrot, cress, watercress, cheese and eggs, or cheese and meat of choice, potato in jacket with a little butter. Use a little safflower or olive oil. Do not have a pudding or sweet. Use dandelion leaves also if you like them.

Supper: This should be taken an hour or so before going to bed. Yogurt with honey, or milk drink. With banana or apple if hungry.

Nothing should be eaten or drunk between these meals, except a fruit juice, or water, if thirsty. If there is a bloated feeling, cut down the quantities.

The full diet
It is very difficult to tell another human being exactly what to eat, and even the diets listed above must only be seen as suggestions. Not only does available money condition what we eat, but also our temperament, glandular balance, and energy expended, produce different needs. Therefore, I can only suggest different principles which you yourself must apply in the way you see fit. Be courageous enough to experiment, and if you are not as healthy as you should be, keep on experimenting until you find the diet that produces the maximum well-being.

1. All food should be as wholesome and unrefined as possible. This means the cutting out of white flour, white sugar, sweets, fried or overcooked foods, all the ready mixed cake mixes, and white flour products, spiced foods and shop pastries.

2. As much food as possible should be eaten raw and fresh, except for eggs, meat and potatoes.

3. Many experts see meat as an unessential part of the diet – – others are the opposite. But pork and the red meats are best

avoided or used infrequently during pregnancy, and always well cooked. If you do eat meat though, make sure to regularly include the organ meats.

4. Have at least one meal each day entirely of fresh, uncooked, and unsugared fruit. This acts as a daily cleansing. No milk, tea, or bread should be taken with this alkaline meal. Milk does not mix well with oranges anyway. In many cases, it is found best to have this meal last thing at night.

5. For the pregnant woman a salad each day repays every effort.

6. Butter is better than the artificial fats, despite all the cholesterol scare. If raw foods, and those low in concentrated starches, are used this is nullified. But make sure a few nuts, wheatgerm, sunflower seeds, or safflower oil is taken daily, or else the vital vitamins F and E are not supplied.

7. Milk is not vital, but if you do not drink a pint or more daily, make sure you get its equivalent in other calcium and protein-rich foods. If you can take yogurt, make your own by beating into a pint of whole milk or dried milk one dessert-spoon of plain yogurt, and stand in a warm place, such as an airing cupboard or vacuum flask, until set.

8. For some women during pregnancy the supplements are the doorway to retaining their baby. In others, the supplements are not essential, but they are a very sound investment. I have personally seen women during pregnancy blossom into glowing health after a few weeks on them. In one case, with a woman who began supplements in her fourth month, the baby was born with a line down its lip. Later a doctor looking at the baby remarked that it had already had an operation to join its hare lip. Of course, no such operation had taken place, but it seems likely that the hare lip was healed while still in the womb through receiving vital nutrients. One medical article, quoted by Carlton Fredericks, says that deficiency of vitamin B$_6$ (found richly in brewer's yeast) can cause the birth of deformed babies. A medical report says that if a woman gives birth to a baby with a hare lip, deformed spine, cleft palate, or club foot, it would be a good thing for her to take vitamin supplements during her *next*

pregnancy! This seems to be a case of telling us to shut the gate after the horse has gone. Thus, at the very least, it is safe insurance to take a daily multi-vitamin and mineral capsule, while it is even better to supply the body's needs adequately. Some doctors argue that high doses of vitamins are toxic, but they fail to point out that this is only true when taken in hundreds of thousands of units. Also, such cases of toxicity are not like the irreparable damage done by most drugs; for if the dose is then stopped, the toxicity disappears.

To repeat the remark made by the mother of a pregnant woman who had not only looked very ill before beginning supplementary vitamins, but who was told by the doctor she would never carry the baby: 'She looks as if she has regained her youth and beauty she had before she was married. All her sickness and symptoms have disappeared, her hair is shining and when the doctor saw her he said, "My goodness, you look well." '

9. We may class as supplements not only vitamins and mineral tablets, but also wheatgerm, molasses, dried milk, brewer's yeast, kelp, Irish moss, garlic tablets, papaya, and Florus.

10. The personal application of the full diet can be built around that given under the Weight Losing Diet.

11. As for exactly what supplements to take: in all cases it is suggested that brewer's yeast, and wheatgerm be added to the diet. A multi-vitamin and mineral supplement,* vitamins C and E, and molasses should be taken. (That is, 100 i.u. of E, and 200 mlg of C, daily.) Also at least six kelp tablets. Otherwise, use particular directions as in health questionnaire, or in following chapter on 'Problems'.

In cases where you feel a little under par, a daily dose of 300 mlg of vitamin C, 200 mlg of vitamin E, and iron and calcium tablets, plus one vitamin and mineral supplement capsule should be taken. Do not feel apprehensive. The girl whose mother's remarks I have mentioned above was on 2,000 mlg

---

* These tablets are obtainable from health food stores, but may not be stocked by chemists. Make sure that any vitamin and mineral supplement has A, B, C, D and E vitamins, and the minerals.

of vitamin E, and the same dose of vitamin C, plus other supplements, gradually reducing.

Just before or during labour, i.e. as labour begins, take 1,000 mlg of vitamin C, four calcium (or six kelp) tablets, and 1,000 i.u. of vitamin E.

12. Virtually all dietary aids, or disciplines, are greatly enhanced by sufficient exercise. This is because the body and its organs need to be stimulated for their best performance and function.

13. Doctors have discovered that too much salt in the diet of a pregnant woman not only causes unnecessary weight gain and restlessness, but also makes birth more difficult. Sufficient salt is in cheese and butter, and should not be used in cooking or on meals.

14. *Please remember, in all cases*, take vitamins E, C, and kelp; one vitamin and mineral capsule, and plenty of brewer's yeast powder and wheatgerm. If you just cannot acquire the taste for brewer's yeast powder, then take the brewer's yeast tablets. Avoid using the extra potency type however, as they upset some people. As I have already said, I think the vitamin A in the vitamin/mineral capsules may be too high for some people. So if headaches, nose bleeds, or itchy skin occur, drop this capsule entirely.

What's in our food?
This part of the chapter is not essential reading, but is included as a more detailed reference for those who need it. It attempts to give a deeper insight into just what each part of food does, so you can use this knowledge to help yourself where necessary.

Food is made up of fats, carbohydrates, proteins, vitamins and minerals. We will therefore look at each of these in turn, and briefly see what part it plays in our health, and in childbearing.

Fats. In our body and in our diet, fats have several essential roles. In our body fatty tissues protect and support vital organs. They act as padding in areas taking much wear, such as fingers. Also, fatty tissues insulate against cold, and act as a reserve food store for when we miss a meal, work harder or breast-feed a baby. In early societies, more subject to the seasonal flux of food, such fat stores were often essential and highly regarded. Possibly sensible reducing diets play the parts of seasonal hunger?

During digestion, proteins can be changed by the liver into fats, sugars and carbohydrates, but fats, sugars and carbohydrates cannot be changed into proteins. Some vitamins such as A are fat soluble, and a fat-free diet endangers the proper absorption of these.

Scientists have found that the reason some babies are born with eczema is that the mother did not have sufficient unsaturated fats in her diet. Inclusion of butter, nuts, olive oil or corn oil in the diet will counteract this.

Carbohydrates. All carbohydrates, such as sweets, biscuits, potatoes, and jam, are turned into sugars during digestion. Starches are made up of chains of sugars linked together. During digestion these chains unlink and return to their basic sugars. While we definitely need a fair amount of carbohydrate in our diet, there are certain dangers, especially if they are taken as concentrated carbohydrates such as white flour, white sugar, ice cream, chocolate, cakes and whips. The digestion and utilisation of starches uses high amounts of vitamin C and the B group of vitamins. In natural starches, such as whole rice or whole wheat, high amounts of these vitamins and minerals occur. When rice or wheat are processed, these nutrients are removed, and so vitamin deficiencies occur. Many people eating a normal amount of vitamin C in their diet suffer from scurvy because their intake of starches and sugar is so high.

This is doubly dangerous because such starches are very filling, and so the appetite is fooled into believing itself satisfied, yet essential minerals and vitamins are missing from one's food intake. Before the motor-car, central heating, ready-made entertainment, and civilisation in general, our forebears had so much exercise that large amounts of starches were burnt up. The large amount of food they thus ate brought a sufficient supply of vitamins and minerals. Lacking this ability to safely consume so much starch, our meals must be planned to include large amounts of minerals and vitamins, with a reasonable amount of starch.

This is why wholewheat flour is advised, and dark brown sugar. If you are going to eat starches, as you must, then at least eat those with very high mineral and vitamin content.

It has been found that a too high carbohydrate diet definitely predisposes one to sinus trouble, catarrh, the common cold, indigestion and poor skin. The section on the alkaline diet suggests a quick cleansing programme. For a woman who has to supply not only her own nutritional needs, but also those of her growing baby, a wise use of starches is essential. The suggestions in the Full Diet will give guidance.

Proteins. All cells are built of protein in some degree. As our body is made entirely of cells, the need for protein is of prime importance. Girls who have skimpy meals of coffee and rolls, which lack protein, soon become ill. Nature makes various proteins out of a mixture of twenty-two acids, called amino acids.

A body lacking sufficient protein, backed by minerals and vitamins, tends to slouch, due to the muscles being weak. Likewise, cracked or peeling nails, brittle hair, poor digestion, low blood-pressure, anaemia and susceptibility to infections, are all traceable to insufficient protein. This is because nail cells, hair, digestive enzymes, artery walls, heart blood cells, and antibodies are all largely protein. If the protein intake is too low, or not supplying all the needed amino acids, these basic body parts function poorly.

The proteins in muscle meats contain fewer of some of the essential amino acids than the organ meats. All animal protein foods such as fish, milk, cheese, meat, and eggs contain all the amino acids. Only egg white is incomplete.

Vegetable proteins, such as brewer's yeast, some nuts, soyabeans, cottonseed, wheatgerm and other cereal germs, also contain all the amino acids, but sometimes in lower quantities than the animal protein foods. However, brewer's yeast, weight for weight, contains more protein than any other food. The amounts of amino acids in brewer's yeast are very near to those in human milk, and the large amounts of B vitamins and minerals it contains make it an extraordinary food. Soyabeans are very high in protein and also contain necessary unsaturated fats or oils.

The lack of one of the amino acids, methionine, is now known to cause swollen ankles in pregnant women. However, the recommended full diet gives a range of complete animal and vegetable proteins.

Vitamins. Next in our list of food constituents come the vitamins. A vitamin is a microscopic substance found in foods, needed by our body for its well-being. Edgar Cayce has said that vitamins are the creative forces working with the body energies for the renewing of the body. By this he meant Life's creative forces; and he also said vitamins are 'that from which the glands take those necessary influences to supply the energies to enable the various organs of the body to reproduce themselves.'

Vitamin A. There is no vitamin A in any fruit or vegetables, only the substance 'carotene' from which our body manufactures the true vitamin. Carotene is found in all green leaves, carrots, tomatoes, pumpkin, prunes, peaches, oranges, cherries, apricots, turnip greens, spinach and in most vegetables. As this is a fat-soluble vitamin, we need fair amounts of fat in our diet to assimilate it, and some people cannot properly convert carotene to vitamin A. Therefore they need it done for them. Animals such as cows, fish, etc., have already converted carotene, and so the fats, such as butter, cream, fish oils and meats, that we get from them are often high in true vitamin A.

This vitamin is used in many ways by the body. One of the first signs that we need more is a dry, rough skin. Goose pimples occur, especially on the thighs, upper arms and back, sometimes causing spots where a hair emerges. Vitamin A is needed for the health of our mucous membranes. These are the soft skin that covers the inside of the nose, mouth, sexual organs, bladder and internal organs. This membrane of skin has the job of keeping at bay millions of bacteria, and uses vitamin A in its germ killing. When the vitamin is insufficient, this defence system breaks down, and infections of nose, mouth and bladder can result. Discharges occur from these areas due to the dying bacteria and cells. Thus colds, bronchitis, catarrh, mouth sores, etc., result.

As vitamin A is used to produce the 'visual purple' in the eyes, another symptom of deficiency is night blindness, sore eyes, the need for sunglassses, or burning eyes. Other signs are teeth cavities, soft bones, bladder stones, and horny skin.

As it is one of the vitamins that can be toxic in too high quantities, an overdose can cause constant headache, nose bleeds, itchy skin and lethargy.

B vitamins. These vitamins have so many functions in the body it is impossible to do more than hint at them here. One of their basic properties is to act as wicks in the body. Using the B vitamins, the body burns the fats and carbohydrates, changing them into energy. Lacking these vitamins, incomplete 'burning' takes place, causing indigestion, furred or strawberry red tongue, constipation, nervousness or depression.

Some of the other members of the B group are: biotin: a deficiency impairs the body's fat production, and may lead to dry skin and lassitude. Choline: essential to health of heart and blood vessels, liver and kidneys. Inositol: reduces liver fats, and stimulates intestinal movements. Thiamin: aids food assimilation, growth, elimination, circulation and heart function. It also plays a part in reducing alcoholism, sciatica, *morning sickness* and *pain*. It is therefore necessary for the pregnant woman to assure sufficient amounts.

Riboflavin: a deficiency causes cracked lips, bald patches on lips, purple tongue, scaly patches around the nose, forehead and eyes, and burning eyes. Niacin: a deficiency causes tender gums, diarrhoea, nausea, insomnia, abdominal pains, and all symptoms linked with depression, melancholy, dizziness. Pyridoxine: deficiency causes pellagra, muscular stiffness, rigidity, hardening of the arteries and tooth decay. It aids digestion of fats, proteins, skin health and nerves, muscle and blood. Pantothenic acid: aids peripheral neuritis, alcoholism, fatigue, breathlessness, fainting spells, and sometimes restores hair to its natural colour. PABA: aids intestinal bacteria to produce folic acid, and a deficiency can produce nervousness, tiredness and depression. Folic acid acts as a preventative to anaemia through promoting red cell growth. Deficiency may cause inflammation of the tongue, gastric troubles, diarrhoea. B_{12}, when deficient, causes pernicious anaemia. It is also used in the treatment of multiple sclerosis, alcoholism, hepatitis and bursitis. It is an antidote to cyanide and lead poisoning.

Nutritionists have said again and again that a deficiency of a single B vitamin is impossible, and so we should never take just one of the vitamins without the others. They are all found in brewer's yeast, in high quantities. Also in peanuts, wholewheat flour, brown rice, salmon, spinach, luna beans, mushrooms, egg yolk, barley, oats, molasses, beef, liver, cheddar cheese, wheatgerm, soyabeans, dandelion leaves and torula yeast.

Vitamin C. This definitely plays the role of strengthening the capillaries, our tiny blood vessels. These minute tubes, when vitamin C is deficient, easily break and cause internal bleeding. Therefore, one of the early signs that we need more of this vitamin is bleeding gums or when we bruise easily. Another of its functions is to unite with poisons in the body and thus counteract them, they are then passed out of the body in the urine. This makes it not only a very efficient antidote to many poisons, but also an infection fighter.

Deficiency also causes poor wound healing, varicose veins, prolonged infections and easy fatigue. Because it strengthens capillaries and tissues, it helps prevent miscarriage. It is useful in the treatment of colds, headaches, migraine, stomach or eye ulcers, burns, cuts, menopause complaints, soft bones, whooping cough and pneumonia. It is also necessary for the proper assimilation of iron, and aids storage of calcium and phosphorus. It should be taken in large quantities in the first stage of labour, as it aids healing, enables one to face stress, gives energy, prevents excess bleeding and helps relaxation.

It is found in large quantities in oranges, lemons, parsley, kale, sprouts, green peppers, blackcurrants, cauliflower, spinach, green lettuce leaves, strawberries, grapefruit, dandelion leaves and onion.

Vitamin D. This vitamin plays a part in the use of calcium in bones and teeth. (Rickets is due to a deficiency.) It is also used to treat psoriasis, tetany, myopia and glandular disturbance. The major source of vitamin D is exposure to sunshine. Our skin oils are changed by sunshine, and are then absorbed into the body again, taking with them vitamin D. If we wash a few hours before or after such exposure, however, the skin oils are washed off, and so no absorption takes place. Vegetable oils rubbed on the skin during sun bathing help to compensate for this though, as long as they too are not washed off too soon.

Other sources are butter, full fat, cheese, full cream yogurt, cream, sunflower seeds, beef, liver, eggs, cod liver or halibut liver – or their oils. It is an essential vitamin for pregnant and nursing mothers.

Vitamin E. Laboratory tests which created a vitamin E deficiency in animals, produced sterility, many miscarriages, still births, wasting of muscles and muscular weakness. Lack of E weakens the hold the placenta has on the wall of the womb.

Vitamin E's function has been found to be to prevent the destruction of essential fatty acids by oxygen. When these fats are oxygenised, they are no longer usable by our body cells. As these fats are vital to each cell, if insufficient essential fatty acids are available, tissue breakdown occurs. This is why muscular wasting occurs during vitamin E deficiency. A lack of vitamin E is a major cause of premature birth. Also hundreds of premature babies have gone blind due to being placed in oxygen tents. As oxygen ruins the essential fatty acids, it causes tissue breakdown in the babies' eyes. Babies who were given vitamin E injections all survived with their sight.

Blood cells are among those that break down due to E deficiency. This causes anaemia in adults and babies. This is why it is a wise precaution for the mother to supplement her diet with vitamin E capsules.

It is interesting that some of the first astronauts suffered anaemia badly after a flight spent breathing richly oxygenated air. Present astronauts have to eat a vitamin E-enriched diet.

Experiments on bulls given vitamin E resulted in a greatly reduced percentage of malformed calves. This is why prospective fathers are advised to take E before trying for a baby.

This vitamin is found in whole wheat, brown rice, peanuts, all whole seeds, nuts, soyabeans, kale, savoy, lettuce, nettle-leaves, peas, cress, and all whole cereals.

Vitamin F. The constituents of this are known as essential fatty acids. They aid the body to get rid of superfluous fat deposits, and in overcoming some skin diseases, such as eczema, boils, psoriasis, etc. They are also important in the treatment of two serious diseases, coeliac and sprue. They play a part in preventing falling hair, dandruff, prostrate disorder and dry skin. Found in whole wheat, wheatgerm, nuts, olive oil, safflower oil, and sunflower seeds. The oils should not be heated however, as this destroys their properties.

Vitamin K. This is largely produced by the intestinal bacteria, except when a person is on antibiotics taken orally. Intestinal bacteria are increased by eating yogurt and raw foods, or Florus. This vitamin is essential for correct blood coagulation. It is thus of great importance to those who frefrequently miscarry. It can be obtained from kale, green cabbage, spinach and nettle leaves – any dark green leaves. It is now general practice to inject this vitamin into newborn babies, to decrease the chance of internal bleeding due to birth.

Vitamin P. Another vitamin aiding prevention of haemorrhaging, and aiding blood coagulation. It occurs in the peel of oranges, but need not be worried about unless used for preventing frequent miscarriages, when it can be taken as bioflavon tablets. If you take vitamin C tablets during pregnancy, buy ones including bio-flavon.

The minerals. These consist of potassium, calcium, iron, hydrogen, oxygen, nitrogen, phosphorus, sulphur, chlorine, iodine, sodium, magnesium, copper, zinc, manganese, vanadium and fluorine. A balanced diet, as suggested in the Full Diet section, will supply all of these in sufficient quantity. Only iron, calcium, phosphorus, sodium, magnesium and sometimes iodine are needed in greater quantities during pregnancy.

Iron. Iron is used in the body largely to make the haemoglobin of the red blood cells. Iron *is* the red of these cells. It is the part of the blood cell that can take hold of oxygen as the blood passes through the lungs, and act as a carrier for the body cells. Therefore, with insufficient iron the oxygen is not carried adequately to the rest of the body from the lungs. Lacking red blood cells, sufferers are usually pale and anaemic. They become easily tired and breathless, having to pant to gain enough oxygen. Also, this leads often to giddiness and depression, fainting and exhaustion.

Iron is found in large quantities in almonds, yeast extracts, beans, brazil nuts, carrageen moss, eggs, dried figs, wholewheat flour, wheatgerm, lentils, molasses, peas, prunes, Barbados sugar, honey, leeks, oats and kelp.

Iron is best absorbed if vitamin C is present in the same meal. Therefore, if taking iron in tablet form, either take C with it, or any of those tablets already containing it.

Calcium. This mineral plays many roles in the body. It is the building material of bones and teeth, regulates heart rhythm, relaxes muscular and nervous tension, helps blood to clot, sometimes helps people underweight to build tissue, and is helpful for insomniacs and some skin disorders.

Calcium is used to form collagen, which is the body tissue that gives firmness to sinews, ligaments, joints and blood flesh. Droopy flesh, weak joints or displaced inernal organs may be due to calcium lack.

The pregnant woman needs a great deal of calcium due to the high quantity used by the baby to build its own bones and tissues. Also, as calcium acts as a muscles and nerve relaxant, it is a really natural sedative at childbirth. For its proper absorption, vitamins A, B, C, and D, especially C, are needed with it. This is why fresh, whole milk is an excellent source.

Other sources are: almonds, soyabeans, carrageen moss, Cheddar cheese, molasses, parsley, spinach, Barbados sugar, kelp, milk products.

Signs of deficiency are muscle cramp, irritability, nervousness, painful periods.

Phosphorus. If you are eating a fair amount of salads and fruit, it is unlikely that you lack this mineral. If you eat a lot of meat and no milk, a calcium *and* phosphorus deficiency may exist. This is true also if a lot of yeast, liver or vitamin B tablets are taken without taking extra calcium. This is because phosphorus works in conjunction with calcium to build bones and teeth, tissues and cartilage. If no calcium is in the meal, the phosphorus passes out into the urine, but combines with blood calcium as it does so, causing a calcium deficiency.

Phosphorus is found in almonds, beans, wholewheat flour, carrageen moss, Cheddar cheese, eggs, yeast extracts, peanuts, peas, walnuts, brewer's yeast and kelp.

Sodium. Apart from anything else, organic sodium (sodium found in vegetables and fruit, not salt) is used by the liver to detoxify the body. This is one of the most 'healing' of activities in the system. Sodium also aids in the right water balance in the body, preventing excess loss of body fluids.

Sources are cucumber, carrots, celery, apples, spinach, and all the squash family such as melons, zuchini, marrow, etc.

Magnesium. Another of the minerals, like calcium and iron, which is often missing in our modern diet. Deficiencies show as tension, muscular cramps or spasms, convulsions. Other symptoms are insomnia, mental confusion, muscular weakness, irregular pulse, shaking hands and twitching.

Babies suffering convulsions and even epilepsy can be

quickly righted by giving magnesium. It is easily available as Epsom salt, and the daily dose in above cases should be about a quarter of a teaspoon. Also it can be bought as Dolomite tablets.

Animals placed on a magnesium-deficient diet quickly developed convulsions, kidney stones, and heart troubles. Magnesium taken in sufficient quantity quickly cures these symptoms, and has been found to decrease cholesterol level dramatically, and cure hardening of the arteries.

People surviving a heart attack and given daily doses of magnesium made 'truly remarkable' progress.

Adelle Davis points out that calcification of tissues, as in arthritis, rheumatism, bursitis, scleroderma, and hardening of the arteries, *does not* mean one should eat less calcium. Improvement can only come, she says, when the calcium and magnesium level are raised.

As magnesium is necessary for calcium metabolism, vitamin C is unusable without it, and it aids in bone formation and relaxing nerves and muscles, so pregnant mothers must ensure an adequate supply. Any high sensitivity to noise, or hand tremors, should be taken as a sign of deficiency.

It is found in almonds, beans, bran, brussels sprouts, chard, clams, nuts, oats, corn, dates, figs, cucumbers, raisins, honey and prunes.

Iodine. This is not frequently deficient except in cases of goitre. Iodised table salt, or the use of kelp tablets, will fulfil the need. It is found in cabbage, carrageen moss, kelp, leeks, lettuce and onions.

Acid and alkali foods. One of the most practical and yet simple pieces of information about foods is their acid and alkaline properties. People have suffered years of discomfort with indigestion or acidity which has been cured in a few days once these principles were understood. Likewise, those suffering from rheumatism, arthritis and sciatica have found either a cure, or great help, from this knowledge. This section is also given to provide greater insight into the use of the cleansing diets mentioned earlier.

Any food we eat produces in our stomach one of three

reactions – acid, alkaline or neutral. This reaction produces a marked influence on the rest of the body, either as a cleansing or clogging influence.

Acid. The following foods tend to be energy-producing and protein foods. These are what we might call the concentrated 'fuel' or 'body building' foods. If we are very active physically, these foods are used and 'burnt up'. If we are not very active, yet eat plenty of these foods, the fuel is not burnt and becomes a clogging and toxifying agent instead. This clogging of the system shows as catarrh, bronchitis, constipation, poor skin, breath odour, and the conditions mentioned above. Part of this is because these foods produce an acid reaction during digestion, and if not burnt up, produce too much acidity in the system as a whole. Any gardener knows that an acid soil needs alkalising; but here are the acid-forming foods:

All fats and oils, prunes, plums, rhubarb, cranberries, all cereals – this includes bread, pastry, cakes, tapioca, custard, pies, etc. Sugar, molasses, sweets, chocolate, all nuts, cream, beans, meat, poultry, fish, potatoes, egg white.

Because meats, sugar and white flour products are particularly irritating to rheumatism and arthritis, many doctors now place such patients on a vegetarian diet.

Alkaline. Many of these foods contain acids, but nevertheless produce an alkaline reaction during digestion. These tend to be the vitamin and mineral foods rather than the body building ones. Although in some people these foods, such as oranges, seem to produce acidity, this is only because the person's system is loaded with too much concentrated starches such as white flour, sugar or meat foods. A few days on the cleansing diet would soon alter this. These foods help to cleanse the system of toxins.

All fruits (except large prunes, plums and rhubarb) are alkaline in digestion.* This includes figs, raisins, dates, sultanas, apples, apricots, blackberries, lemons, oranges, etc. Also all vegetables, such as sprouts, lettuce, carrots, cucum-

* But only in normally functioning digestions. Sufferers from acute arthritis and rheumatism are advised to avoid such 'acid' fruits as grapefruits and lemons.

ber, young peas, runner beans – but not broad beans, processed peas, dried beans, etc., or when cooked in oil or fat.

Neutral. A few foods are neutral in reaction. These are brown rice, honey, buttermilk, yogurt, cream cheeses and banana.

As can be seen from all that has been said in this chapter, some foods, such as almonds, yogurt, molasses, brewer's yeast and uncooked fruits and vegetables, have so many advantages that it is wise to include them in our daily diet. In the case of brewer's yeast and molasses, this can be done by adding them to our cooking, such as in our homemade bread or cakes. Or with yogurt, a banana and honey, placed in a blender with yogurt, produces a delicious drink.

4.

Breathing In and Out of Labour

Everything that we do involves our whole being. But of course, different activities alter the balance between the parts of our total self. For instance, if I am swimming, some of the blood may have been taken away from the digestive tract to be circulated in the voluntary muscles. Thus the rate of digestion may be slowed but the activity of the muscles, heart, and lungs greatly increased. While swimming I am probably not thinking deeply, or aware of finer emotional feelings not connected with the physical sensations of the water. On the other hand, if I am sitting reading, my digestion can go ahead undisturbed, I am probably little aware of my physical sensations if the book is interesting, but am much more alive to the world of thought, memory, emotion and comparison. In fact, different activities concentrate our awareness on the various parts of our being; as in sleep, where what remains of consciousness contacts parts of self usually right outside our range of awareness.

Unconscious tensions and fears
If we carry this illustration farther, it also becomes obvious that habits we have formed in the past, often quite unconsciously, largely control situations in the present. For instance, my wife was nearly drowned as a young girl, and now has a dread of swimming. Because of this her emotional reaction to the water creates physical tension and timidness, making it difficult to trust her body to it. Of course, such habit patterns can be changed and gradually replaced by new ones. To do this, however, often requires us to become very

conscious of the old habit and what it is doing to our body and emotions. A friend who once broke a bone in his foot, because of the pain, learnt to walk on the side of his foot, and still carried on walking this way years later, even though the break had healed perfectly. But many of the things that hurt us are not physical. As a child or even as an adult, someone we love and trust may have badly hurt us, and without realising it we withdraw our feelings in order not to be hurt again. Just as my wife cannot trust her body to water because of her original terror, so we, if hurt in love, may also find it difficult to once again trust our own feelings to the intimate relationship of sharing ourselves deeply with someone else. I wish to stress again that we may be quite unaware of this.

We have already seen how such unconscious tensions or fears may cause us to take on a posture of withdrawal or tenseness during intercourse or childbirth. If you are now wondering what all this has got to do with breathing and giving birth, it is simply that I am trying to show how all these different aspects of life are linked. Also, just as when the actual birth occurs, all that we have done in the way of exercises, diet, relaxation and development of helpful habit patterns, is all brought together in the one event, so in our actual study and practice I do not wish you to lose sight of the unity of these different things. After all, while you are having the baby, you obviously do not want to have the bother of directing attention from relaxing the back, to correct breathing, to surrendering, to relaxing the face, and so on. Better to have one routine that covers the lot, than a method so complex it becomes impractical. In describing it however, a chapter is devoted to each aspect of the one routine to explain it more adequately. In any case, in our hurried world, who is going to have time to practise all these different techniques? Therefore we must attempt to incorporate each with the other.

The need for air
Before such incorporation can take place, we have to be

breathing correctly. The habits arising out of emotional tension influence many people's breathing patterns and have to be corrected before proceeding on to further methods. This is important, as faulty breathing cannot help but place a strain on the body, especially that of the pregnant woman. Many people tend to forget the body's enormous need for oxygen, and that the baby breathes through the mother's lungs. To indicate the importance of air to the body and soul (for breathing influences consciousness), there is an ancient and much quoted yoga statement, which says that while we can go without food for weeks and yet remain alive, or without water for days, we can only go without air for a few minutes. In another way we can get a similar picture of the need for air. During each day we may drink about a quart or more of liquid; we may eat several pounds in weight of food; but in the same period we breathe in about 375 cubic feet of air.

As far as science is concerned, oxygen combines with carbon in the body cells and forms carbon dioxide. This union produces heat and energy. If the supply of oxygen is cut off to particular cells, the flame of life literally goes out in them. If it is reduced below their needs, they are made to function inadequately. Yoga, and some aspects of modern research, such as that done by Dr Reich, also see the breathing rhythm as an expression of life itself. Reich has postulated a cosmic energy radiating from the sun, which he named 'orgone', which when acting upon matter expresses its innate qualities by producing our form, movement, and consciousness. One of the basic movements expressed when this cosmic energy activates a physical form is pulsation, or contraction and expansion, tension and relaxation. This we see in the spontaneous sexual movements already discussed; also in breathing, and childbirth. Every spontaneous movement is in fact an expression of this relationship between what yoga calls prana, and Reich calls orgone, and the body. Heartbeats and breathing are particularly good examples of this.

If this idea is difficult to grasp, and it seems hard to understand how an energy can cause spontaneous physical movements, insight might be gained by thinking about a simple example. I believe everybody must have had the experience of hearing a pin, or other small object, vibrate in a vase, or on a shelf, when a particular note or sound is made either on the television or by passing traffic. Particles of sand on a piece of stretched cellophane will also vibrate when we sing or speak near it. This is how the telephone works. If we realise that our body is a very complex receiving instrument, and can be made to respond in the most amazing ways to the sea of energy in which we live, this is a very basic idea of the yoga philosophy regarding the cause of existence. But while the example of a pin bathed in the sea of energy we call sound, and sometimes moved by it when there is resonance between pin and sound, helps us to understand the resonance between our physical form and the energy which enlivens it, yet something remains unexplained. It is that the pin has no choice as to whether it will surrender to the spontaneous movement, or fight against it through fear, habit, or self will. As, in our case, consciousness and decision, or will, are produced by energy interacting with matter, we can interfere with the instinctive patterns of expression that arise in us.

It is strange that the thing created, even though it depends utterly upon its source, can yet interfere with that which creates it. This opens up the possibility of seriously injuring the natural function of creative on created. In other words, it is like a car destroying some of its wiring or turning the ignition control, and thus advancing or retarding the ignition, and putting the engine out of tune. As far as yoga is concerned, this is the major cause of misery in our life. Knowingly or unknowingly our will has been directed against that which creates us, causing it to misfunction in our being. (I would like to point out for those who are thinkers with scientific background, this explanation is only analogical. Yoga does not separate matter and energy, or matter, energy, and mind. It does see that what we call energy interacts with what we call matter, but it points out that these are merely polarities of a single thing – just as the left hand can interact with the right hand, yet are one and the same body.)

As I hope you will begin to see, the golden thread of this book is to give methods which will help you to find your natural, spontaneous source of health, love and life. Throughout the book the attempt is made to let go of those habits and fears that are acting against your own innate nature. This chapter on breathing follows the same aim. Although in theory it is sufficient to surrender our will, habits and fears to the natural and spontaneous workings of our being, in practice we often need to help the process along. We do not need to look for the reason. It is that many of our fears or habits are so deep rooted or unconscious, that we cannot let go of them even when we decide to. This is because we no longer have hold of *them* – they have hold of *us*. Thus, a man who, despite the fact he loves his wife and has decided to be faithful, yet allies with several other women, does so because despite his decision, his passions have too strong a hold on him.

Analysis of our breathing pattern
Therefore, before we can integrate our breathing practice into the exercise routine already given, we need to view the overall pattern of our breathing, and maybe help it into line a little. To analyse our own breathing pattern, a simple method can be used. Sit in a chair, or kneel on a yoga blanket, hips on heels, back straight. Put one hand on chest, one on solar plexus, just breathe in as far as possible without letting the chest rise. If this is successful the hand on the solar plexus will rise, without the one on the chest moving much at all. A point will be reached in the inhalation where you cannot breathe in any more without moving the hand on the chest. At this point allow the chest to rise until full inhalation is reached. As this happens the hand on the solar plexus will probably drop back a little. This is quite normal. If your pregnancy is fairly well advanced there will be less ability to raise the solar plexus hand first, but there should still be some ability to do so.

This little test shows us whether we have the natural cycle

of abdominal breathing. If you cannot breathe in and raise the solar plexus hand first, then wrong habits or tensions are interfering with normal breathing. The fact that the abdomen does not rise shows that your breathing is also inadequate, and the lungs are not being sufficiently filled with air. This will obviously decrease the amount of oxygen available within the lungs – and, just as important, the waste products that pass out of the body via the lungs will not be properly eliminated. This is a sort of thoracic constipation. During pregnancy it is more important than ever to make sure that our elimination from the lungs is sufficient, as the baby also eliminates some of its own poisons through the mother's lungs. We do not have to be fanatical about this; but we do have a goal in view, that of helping 'nature' to produce a beautiful and healthy child. Efficient breathing is part of the activities that together mould and form the baby.

Another test for tensions
Another test to determine how much our own breathing pattern is controlled or disrupted by tension is as follows: Sit or kneel as before. Take a slow deep breath in. Now breathe out rapidly until the lungs are as empty as possible. If this outbreathing is in one unbroken stream from 'full' to 'empty', then all is well. Many people will find however, that try as they may, they cannot exhale in an unbroken stream. There will be 'catches' where they stop for a moment and then continue. Clinical work done by a number of therapists has shown that this disturbed exhalation is a sign that the person is controlled by a fear, resulting in tension. Such tension not only influences the breathing of the person, but also the relationship with other people, and events in life. This usually produces un-satisfactory sex life, and other emotional or life problems. Because we are concentrating there only on yoga as it directly relates to pregnancy we cannot go into a long description of how to deal with such problems in detail. But at least a general method must be given because such tensions usually cause unnecessary difficulties during confinement.

The following breathing methods are not necessary for

those whose breathing cycle is normal. They are recommended for those who, in the above tests, found that their natural breathing was interfered with. If you found that you could not breathe abdominally and move the solar plexus hand, it is sufficient to frequently practise the movement until it is attained. The aim is to make proper abdominal breathing into a habit. This will require persistence and patience. Our ingrained habits arise because we have performed the activity hour after hour. In the attempt to breathe correctly we not only have to instil in ourselves the correct pattern, but we also have to eradicate the old method.

Methods
Therefore, if you do not breathe abdominally, for ten minutes after the postures sit or lie comfortably, one hand on the chest, one on the solar plexus. Breathing slowly and fully, try to breathe raising the lower hand first as already described. Keep steadily at this for ten minutes, and keep at it each day until you eventually learn how to do it. Once you get the hang of it, you can naturally dispense with the use of the hands. Also, once the method is established, concentrate on it at odd moments of the day, such as while out walking. In this case breathe in and out in time with your strides. For instance three strides breathing in, three strides breathing out – or whatever is easiest for you. By concentrating on it frequently like this, it will quickly become a habit.

If you are unable to breathe out in one smooth flow, the recommended exercise is as follows: Sit upright in a chair, or cross-legged on the floor, or kneel on the floor with the hips on the heels. Breathe in slowly and deeply, hold for a moment and breathe out quickly with a rush through the nose. Breathe slowly in again and repeat. The aim is to gradually break down the resistance that stops the smooth exhalation. This resistance may be an emotional one. For instance, crying causes us to breathe out fully, and if the suppression of grief has caused us this tension then if we break through we will release a lot of grief and weeping. Of course, it may be other fears or suppressed emotions that are behind the faulty breathing. If these arise during the breathing we have to have the courage to let them out and express them.

This is a very stimulating exercise, and it is difficult to give a general length of time to practise it. This is because some people may become slightly dizzy due to the amount of oxygen absorbed. Therefore, you will have to experiment to find your own level. I would suggest at least fifteen repetitions, and not more than one hundred. Practise it daily until the breakthrough to normal expiration occurs. Then, if abdominal breathing is possible, pass on to the ordinary breathing practices mentioned later. Otherwise practise abdominal breathing. If your breathing is abdominal, with a steady exhalation, only general breathing methods need be practised. I stress particularly the importance of deep rhythmic breathing while walking as already described.

For hundreds of years yoga has taught a variety of breathing practices. Some of these are aimed at calming and stilling the mind, others at cleansing the body, others at oxygenating the cells. During childbirth one of the greatest needs is to keep the muscles of the uterus well supplied with oxygen so that it does not become exhausted under the pressure of work. Also, the baby itself may develop an enormous oxygen debt unless the breathing is sufficient during the birth. I am indebted to Erna Wright's description of how psycho-prophylaxis uses breathing methods during childbirth. I have attempted to describe here how to use the traditional yoga methods however, although it must be admitted that as far as I can see it is psycho-prophylaxis that has had the genius to pioneer the use of these practices.

Just as a man who is walking and suddenly starts running will immediately need more oxygen, so in childbirth there are different levels of needs as the body contracts and relaxes. If we completely expressed our instincts, we might pant as a dog does, when contraction occurs. However, being often out of harmony with our instincts it is a wise insurance to prepare ourselves through training, to meet the need as it arises. The following breathing practice should therefore be done every day while relaxing. This should be done whether you have perfected abdominal breathing or not.

Take up your position of relaxation. Begin your relaxation as described in the chapter dealing with it. When you reach the point of tensing parts of the body and at the same time relaxing the rest of the body, incorporate the following: Before you begin the contraction breathe fully but slowly as in the abdominal breathing method. After three or four breaths say to yourself mentally 'contraction beginning'. Now gently contract both arms, relaxing all the rest of the body. As you do this begin the following breathing method. Breathe in through the nose as in the abdominal breathing, but when it comes to breathing out, blow out through the mouth just strongly enough to make a blowing noise. Take three breaths in this way, then tense the arms as hard as possible by bringing the hands to the shoulders as when tensing the biceps. As you do this go into the next stage of breathing. Imagine you are a dog panting. Breathe in and out through the mouth, blowing as you breathe out, to make the characteristic panting noise. This is approximately one out breath per second. Hold the tension and carry on breathing in this way for ten seconds, which is stage three breathing. The others are stage one and stage two, respectively.

At the end of the ten breaths in stage three, relax the arm tension slightly and drop into stage two breathing for three breaths. After this relax the arms and entire body, and drop into stage one breathing, at the same time saying mentally, 'contraction finished'.

It is fairly obvious that what is being attempted here is to perfect the ability to change the breathing rate at will according to the need of the moment, and at the same time be able to relax all of the body not being contracted. This will undoubtedly seem extraordinarily complicated at first, but practising each session will gradually perfect it so that 'on the day' you will be adept at it. When you have taken three or four breaths in stage one go through the whole procedure again, but this time tense the right arm and left leg instead of both arms. Obviously, at the same time you must keep all the rest of the body relaxed.

After having repeated the cycle using right arm and left leg, go through it one more time using left arm and right leg. When this is finished carry on with the relaxation as described.

When you first start this practice of relaxation and breathing, not only will it seem very complicated, as already said, but it will also take a long time to pass through the various stages of relaxation as described. After a few weeks, however, you will find that the strange ideas are becoming meaningful, the routine is becoming second nature and the whole thing will take far less time. But as a whole it should take at least half an hour.

Erna Wright gives a much more complex method, which I am sure in general is very necessary to achieve the pain-free birth aimed at. Noting the tremendous difference that diet and supplementation makes on the length and progress of birth it is unnecessary to go to such lengths, if the diet given is followed. Many women have a problem-free birth simply through taking the dietary supplements of C, E and calcium. My own wife, during her last pregnancy and eating largely a raw-food diet, practising the yoga postures and taking vitamin supplements, was only three-quarters of an hour in labour. Therefore, as long as the diet suggested is being used, far less discipline need be applied in these other ways, as the vitamin E alone aids oxygenation of tissues, the calcium decreases pain, and the C increases energy level and recuperation. In a later chapter, more details will be given as to how you use the breathing stages on the actual day. Meanwhile, once you have really established the breathing method, after about two months of practice, they need only be practised once each week.

5.

Relaxation and You

A mother of two children once told me the fascinating story of her youngest son's birth. The birth was proving to be very difficult, so much so that she felt she could not go on any longer. Her contractions were such agony that she could bear it no more, and, as it were, she inwardly collapsed. To her amazement, what had been pain became a feeling of great bliss. She said that a most wild and wonderful emotion came upon her. No longer any pain, but like the mounting pleasure of sexual abandon during intercourse, and her son was born in her ecstasy of orgasm.

Think upon this deeply and often, for here is surely the birthright of every woman. Such a moment of creation should not be one of pain, or of discomfort, but of ecstasy. Yet why has it so often been otherwise? Is the answer not in the mother's own description? Only when she collapsed into relaxation, and had thus totally surrendered herself to the process of life taking place, did the ecstasy occur. The previous pain had been due to her unconscious resistance. Yoga, Taoism, Christian mysticism, Zen, Sufism, Judo, and many other schools, have taught for thousands of years that most of man's pain is because he resists Life, resists his own nature, destroys his own natural relationship with his own being.

However, let us be frank with each other. I am a man. I have never given birth to a child. I am only passing on to you the experience of other women. On the other hand, I have used these principles in my own life and seen what were pains in my emotional life become pleasures. I have not found perfect bliss, only an emerging maturity and pleasure in life. You who are reading this book are undoubtedly as much of an imperfect woman as I am an imperfect man. You too must have fears and tensions that create problems and unhappiness in your life as much as I have in mine – maybe less, maybe more. No doubt such inbuilt parts of one's personality may not change overnight, and you may recognise that. You therefore say to yourself, 'What point is there in my practising these methods? How much good will they do me in such a short time?'

You have to bring these questions to the surface and deal with them. Because if you do not they will undoubtedly be there inside you, interfering with the definite benefit you can obtain. My answers to these questions are quite simple. As I have said, I have not found perfect happiness, but I have found a degree of change that is satisfying. Even if a *perfect* childbirth did not result, at least you can achieve satisfying benefits, even in a short time.

On the other hand, I wish to lay particular importance on one thing. The woman I mentioned had practised no preparatory method at all, yet she experienced the secret wonder of birth. I am trying to press you with the fact that you cannot know beforehand just how wonderfully successful you may be when the actual event occurs. Why? Because there is something in men and women which directs their conscious life. You can call it your Source, God, Superconscious, Self – but these are only words. Nevertheless, it has been the experience of people in all races and times that if they but relaxed their own will, fears, and desires, and gave themselves to this unknown factor in their life with open arms and heart, their faltering efforts were often made magnificent.

Co-operate with Life working in you
We have already, step by step, outlined the various blockages, such as in your breathing or genital tension, and shown how habits of relaxed and spontaneous feeling and activity can be cultivated. What I have said about resisting Life's processes active in our being resulting as pain, and co-operation result-

ing as pleasure, shows once more how necessary these habits are for pleasurable childbirth. Earlier, in dealing with yoga postures, it was said that it is the uterus itself, not the abdominal muscles, which expel the baby. It was also said that we cannot directly exercise the muscles of the uterus as we can exercise the other muscles of our body. However, the Life processes we mentioned above do this for us in two ways. Firstly, when our body is well nourished and exercised generally, the tone and quality of muscles that are not directly used in the exercise is increased. This is because any single part of the body cannot help but partake of the standard of health of the body as a whole. Secondly, as the pregnancy advances, the uterus begins to 'practise' for the event. It does this by subtle contractions during the latter part of pregnancy. Many women do not notice these contractions, but if you watch carefully they will soon become obvious. One of the signs is that the abdomen becomes hard and taut. Another is the actual sensation of the uterus flexing itself.

It is around this natural fact that our method of relaxation during the actual birth will be built. For this reason I will point out certain things about it necessary to understand. A method called the 'psycho-prophylactic' technique of childbirth has been developed around becoming conscious of these pre-birth contractions. This was originated in Russia, became popular in France, and is now used by many practitioners. The aim is to have the woman realise that these contractions, which are exactly like birth contractions, are not painful. Of course, these contractions are not as frequent as those at birth, nor are they pushing the baby out through the birth canal. But through becoming aware of them, you can become assured that the contractions are not painful. The pain arises from resistance to the passing of the baby through the passage out of the uterus commonly known as the birth canal; or through muscular cramp due to insufficient calcium. Such resistance is called 'genital tension' during the actual contraction. This naturally stops the baby passing out quickly and easily. Here is a classical example of how our own tensions and fears can interfere with or block a

'Life process', thus causing pain. Therefore, our relaxation method will be entirely aimed at making you capable of relaxation during contraction, and developing the ability to co-operate with Life working in you.

Replace tension with relaxation

You are already learning this during the practices used with the postures. Now, during the relaxation we will take it much deeper. Therefore, after finishing your postures and any breathing practice, lie on your exercise blanket, arms at sides, knees drawn up. Make sure you are warm enough and out of any draught. The idea is to get used to the feeling of muscular contraction, and to build the habit of 'going along with' spontaneous body processes. As this is done, relaxation of all muscles and emotions not involved in the contraction or movement has to take place. Therefore we have to first learn what relaxation is. Technically it is the letting-go of all tension. In practice it is also the dropping of all personal conscious effort and resistance. It can be summed up in the words *surrender* and *co-operation*. Like anything else, if we do not have the ability to relax as a natural talent, we have to learn it, and some people are better at it than others.

Not only do we have to learn what relaxation is, but we also have to learn what tension is. By this I mean that very often we have not learnt to recognise the sensation of tension or relaxation in our body. Not being aware of these states, we may not realise that parts of our body are always tense, or how to drop this tension. Therefore our first step is to practise producing tension and relaxation at will. So, as you are resting on your blanket, with a small pillow under the hollow of your back if necessary, tense as much of your body as you can. You may find it helps to press your feet on the floor, clench your fists, bite your teeth together, and wrinkle your forehead. But make your body as tense as possible. This is muscular tension. Become aware of how it feels. Then slowly drop all the effort and allow your whole body to become loose and limp. Quickly pass your attention up your body to make sure all parts have dropped their effort.

Particularly notice genitals, abdomen, neck, jaw, and forehead. Notice the feeling of relaxation.

Now tense your whole body again, but this time only half as much as before. Then slowly relax, passing the attention quickly over the body. Tense again, but this time so that there is only the *feeling* of tension; hardly a muscle moving. Drop the feeling of tension so the feeling of relaxation can replace it. Pass your attention once more over the body, making sure it is relaxed, and then bring your attention to your arms. Bring your hands up, fists clenched, to touch your shoulders, and tense all the muscles in your arms as hard as you can; but not so hard you cannot hold it for some time. (If your muscles cramp while you are tensing them it is probably because you need more calcium in your diet. So increase your intake of milk, yogurt, or bone meal tablets, or kelp or calcium tablets. Calcium is best absorbed if vitamin D is present, either in the tablet or as cod liver oil.)

Now, while your arms are tense, pass your attention quickly over the rest of the body making sure it is all relaxed. Include the face and neck in the survey. If you have just begun the practice of this relaxation, include the breathing method described at the end of the last chapter. That is, practising breathing in the three levels. Then slowly relax the arms, rest for a while and repeat it twice more. If you have reached the point in pregnancy where you are aware of uterine contractions, then practise your relaxation while such a contraction occurs using the three breathing levels. Become as aware of it as possible, and relax all other parts of the body. The arms are being used as a substitute for contractions of the uterus, to enable you to relax all other parts of the body during contractions. Contraction of one part of the body should not involve contraction of other parts not being used, but with many of us it does.

The next and final stage of the relaxation is a difficult one to induce artificially. As you can see, the first stage was to learn relaxation and tension; the second stage to enable you to maintain relaxation during contraction; and this third stage is an attempt to learn surrender or co-operation with a spontaneous movement or Life process, such as birth is. One of the few ways in which we can learn this outside of the actual event, apart from going along with pre-birth contractions, is as follows: After tensing the arms, rest for a moment until the arms feel normal, and then concentrate your attention on your breathing. Notice the rise and fall of your chest, but do not let your attention interfere with the natural cycle and movement of your breathing. If your attention wanders, bring it back, if necessary, time and time again. After about a minute, just as your inhalation has reached its peak, consciously interfere with your breathing by holding your breath. As you are doing this, watch your sensations intently. Soon an urge or desire to breathe out will arise. Resist it and see the feelings of discomfort begin to increase. If you continued this resistance the feelings of discomfort would soon become acute pain. When the discomfort is obvious, relax your resistance and let the breathing become normal. Make sure once more that your body is relaxed and return your attention to your breathing. This time, as you have breathed out, hold your breath again for a time, then continue breathing; relax the body and return attention to breathing.

In doing this, it can be directly seen that discomfort and then pain is a direct result of interfering with a Life process. We are, of course, here interfering consciously and on purpose. In many cases where we interfere with the innate processes of our being, it is done unintentionally and without realising it. It can also be seen that when we drop our interference, the discomfort disappears and the process continues. In childbirth most discomfort and pain is the result of a similar process. Unconscious tension interferes with the birth process. Or else, the feeling of internal stretching, which would have been only discomfort, has become a pain because the discomfort was resisted by tension and fear. This method of relaxation is to make you very aware of (*a*) interfering with a natural process, and (*b*) relaxing the interference and allowing the process to continue. But we have to take this a stage farther, the reason for this next stage being that most tension in childbirth is due to unconscious fears or habits of tense reaction to discomfort. But what exactly do I mean by that? I have already mentioned my wife's experience of being nearly drowned, and the fact that she now dislikes water. Some people may dread going on boats, or in water, and not know why. If the dread was caused by a babyhood experience of being submerged in bath water, which incident they cannot remember, this is an example of an unconscious fear. It is a fear that arises from factors outside of our present remembrance.

As for 'tense reaction to discomfort', this is like the person with a rotten and painful tooth being unwilling to pass through the discomfort and suffering of having the tooth removed. They thus endure the more prolonged pain of its aching. So it is that sometimes, by withholding or tensing against the discomfort of stretching, it is turned into a pain. Therefore our relaxation aims at developing the ability to let go of our fears and habits, and so allow the process to continue unhampered. To do this we have to be able to surrender, or relax, our whole being. This process has been started in your practice of the postures.

The Life process which causes you to be
Our next step, after interfering with our breathing and then dropping this interference, should thus be as follows. Keep your attention concentrated on the process of your breathing without any interference whatsoever. Realise that 'something' of which you are not aware is causing this activity of your chest. We will simply call this the *Life process which causes you to be* . . . in short, Life.

If this is to be successful, you must make such thoughts very clear and real to yourself. Really think about the subject. Realise now that your heartbeat, digestion, and recuperation are all expressions of this same Life. While relaxing, dwell for a few moments on the thought that your whole body, and the forming body of the baby, is due to Life.

These realisations have to be thought out slowly at first, and step by step, to lead us where we wish to get. The next step after considering your body and its functions as an expression of Life is to turn your attention away from your breathing, to your *self* – your own awareness. Despite the fact that nothing seems as real as our own existence, when we actually attempt to look at self, nothing is more difficult, or seems more obscure. However, we are not attempting higher metaphysical analysis here, we are dealing with the very practical subject of spontaneous childbirth – the healthy, happy process of all your being working harmoniously and pleasurably together to produce your baby. So in looking at self, all I am asking is for you to realise that your very awareness as a conscious being is also the result of Life, just as your breathing and digestion are.

Having seen that you would not exist outside of this *something*, this *process* we have called Life, realise that it holds within itself the very wisdom of what you are. It is you. Therefore, not only does it have the wisdom but also the fantastic power that has caused us to exist. Yet this wisdom, this power, may be quite unknown to us – quite unconscious. In fact, it may only become conscious as we become aware of it, or discover it, in our own life and being.

Don't worry if this seems very complex at present. Do not be concerned if you cannot understand some of it. Take what you can grasp, and pass on. The rest should be allowed to rise gradually. Meanwhile simply put it to one side if it does not make sense to you.

Despite the fact that your body and awareness of yourself, all your functions in fact, have been brought into existence by the unconscious power and wisdom of Life, and thus you are totally dependent upon it, yet you have a relationship with it, not being merely a puppet. You have already seen how you can interfere with your breathing. This is a simple example indeed of how you can impose your will upon Life. But everything you do is influencing what is, after all, your innate being. Your actions either enhance or subdue, aid to unfold or repress its qualities, conflict or co-operate with your own being. For instance, what you eat either supplies or denies the needs of this process you are. What we think or feel either express and satisfy its energies and wisdom, or twist them into dissatisfaction and pain – and so on through our whole life. Religion presents you with the question: 'Are you for or against God?' Yoga asks a different question: 'Are you for or against yourself?' For if we live in conflict with the very process which *is* our own being, we are against ourself and suffer the consequences.

What is Life?
Having come this far we are near the end of our journey. We have seen something of Life and our relationship with it. But what is it?

This is a very important question for a number of reasons. It is obvious from what has already been said that our aim is to not only surrender but to actively co-operate with Life in the search for a spontaneous childbirth. (The term 'spontaneous childbirth' is used to denote a pleasurable birth due to all parts of one's being co-operating.) Therefore we have to know what we are co-operating with. Many people give up their relaxation practice in discouragement because they have never been able to define this very question. This discouragement is undoubtedly due to their expectation of the wrong things. The resulting disappointment is a natural deterrent. Therefore, to avoid the disappointment, let us make sure you are on firm ground, in firm contact, with that which constitutes you. Or at least, let us make sure your expectations are aimed at practical issues.

Basically there are just two ways of realising Life. One is by realising the *results* of its activity. Thus, when we experience our spontaneous breathing or childbirth or consciousness, we are knowing the results of its working. The other way is by *being* it. That is, by there being no differentiation between consciousness and that which produces it. This is yoga, or union between Life and that which arises from it.

For the practical purposes of our relaxation, however, the method of knowing it through its results is sufficient. The last stage of our relaxation therefore resolves itself as follows: Having watched your breathing, held it in, and then relaxed your interference and body; having watched your breathing and seen it as an expression of Life, and realised that you would not exist without it; having seen that nevertheless you have a relationship with it of co-operation or denial – then decide to surrender your whole being to its own natural processes, so that any unconscious or conscious interferences may be smoothed away and harmony result. Do this by letting go, by dropping any ideas, attitudes, prejudices, you may have. While doing this hold the attention on your face and head. Allow any facial tensions or expressions to slip away. Bringing the attention to the chest, let go of any emotions of fear, anger, hate, worry, or in fact any emotions, even of affection, love. Let go of all. Now relax the genitals and let go of your hold on your sexual feelings.

Simply rest now for some minutes in the general feeling of relaxation. *Make a mental picture of the line of light passing through your body and irradiating every part of it. Let yourself go into this light which is a symbol of Life, meanwhile repeating mentally, 'Surrender to Life.'* Say it over and over, bring your attention back if it wanders, time and time again. If restlessness, emotions, tremblings, crying, or worries come up, do not attempt to push them aside or resist them. This only leads to struggle and internal fight. Just let them happen. On the other hand, do not let them stop the period of relaxation. Let them come up and out, but watch them as if you were standing to one side watching somebody else struggle. Realise that they are things happening to you – they are not you! The real you is the thing that experiences all this multitude of changing thoughts and feelings. If you believe your emotions are you, they will carry you away like a twig in a swirling stream. But if you see them simply as events you are experiencing, they lose their control of you.

The relaxation should be practised every day. It may be best done just before getting into bed, as this is the one time of day there is always opportunity to do it, as you can always go to bed a few minutes later. The aim is to get the habit so established that you can easily use the 'handing over' or relaxation during the baby's birth. The frequent practice will also help to free you of inbuilt tensions and problems before the big event occurs. As I have already said, do not expect perfection of yourself. Even our imperfect handing over can still allow that wisdom and power which creates us to help us and lead us harmoniously through the birth. You learn to notice whether you are interfering or co-operating with the activities that arise from Life, which readies you for spontaneous childbirth, wherein your conscious self co-operates with the unknown forces of your being in this wonder of creation.

The method of relaxation
For easy reference we will list the method of relaxation point by point:
1. Make yourself comfortable on your exercise blanket, or in an easy chair. Make sure you are warm enough.
2. Tense your whole body as hard as possible. Slowly relax. Pass your attention over your body relaxing each part, particularly the forehead, jaw, neck, abdomen and genitals.
3. Tense your whole body once more, but this time only half as much as before. Slowly relax and pass the attention over the body as before.
4. Tense the whole body once more, but so slightly that there is only the *feeling* of tension. Release it until there is the *feeling* of relaxation. Again pass the attention over the body.
5. Bring the attention to the arms. Clench the fists and bring the hands to the shoulders, tensing all the muscles in the arms. As you hold this tension in the arms relax all the other parts of the body, and practise the breathing method of using the breath levels. If you are near the end of term and have a uterine contraction, use this instead of the arms. That is, relax the whole body while the uterus contracts.
6. Concentrate your attention on your breathing without interfering. After about a minute, hold your breath in until it becomes uncomfortable. Release it and let the breathing become normal. Make sure your body is relaxed, then do the same, holding the breath out. When uncomfortable, allow normal breathing to continue.
7. As you watch your breathing, realise it is an expression of the *Life process which causes you to be.*

8. Realise that your whole being, body, and mind, and forming baby, are entirely results of Life, and your relationship with it.

9. Realise that you relate to Life either in a co-operative or negative manner.

10. Decide to co-operate with your own innate being, and surrender thinking, emotions, and passions, by letting go of them. Then visualise the light filling your body, and you handing over to it, meanwhile repeating mentally: 'Surrender to Life'.

Relaxation is more than just a practice of lying and tensing one's body and then dropping the tensions. I believe this becomes obvious from what has already been said. Relaxation is also living and acting in accordance with one's own being. But before we leave this subject, I would like to go a little farther into some of the issues raised.

We have postulated for instance that whatever it is, whatever factor or factors causes us to exist, we depend upon it. We have also said that this results in something of an innate being. As an example, a rose weed would find it difficult to grow into a dandelion. It is innately a rose. All the forces in the seed conspire to produce a rose. Similarly, we have certain innate directions, and if we frustrate them we suffer inner conflict and dissatisfaction. We cannot say, however, that everybody's inner directions are the same. So we cannot form a set of rules all must follow, and create a new religious dogma. We can only say that it seems necessary to discover one's own innate needs and direction and attempt to comply with them. It appears as a logical conclusion that this is the only way we can be whole people, at peace with ourselves and the world. For if we are at odds with our own nature, we are more than likely to be at odds with others. The method we have given of relaxation is just one of the ways we can attempt to find unity within ourselves. As a mother-to-be it is essential to seek this unity between the known and unknown parts of your nature; between the voluntary and involuntary parts of your being, because much of birth depends upon the efficient working of involuntary muscles, on chemical changes, glandular activity, and so on. These are all parts of your being you may be at odds with due to tensions, fears, personality traits, and attitudes. As parenthood is also a creative process, an expression of forces that have exteriorised your own body, you can similarly co-operate or disrupt these creative processes.

Needs and deprivations

You may consider such points arguable, and I am not denying you the right to disagree. One thing, however, that I believe most of us have to accept is the innate needs of the body, even if we will not admit the innate needs of the soul and spirit. Our experience with holding the breath is an immediate demonstration of the body's innate need for air. But some of the body's needs are not as immediately noticeable as this. The same applies of course to our innate emotional, mental and spiritual needs. Our needs in these directions, unless they cry out to us as savagely as our need for air, may easily be ignored. But it is true that some of these subtle needs do cry out. After all, our need for air is barely noticeable during the day and night unless we interfere, or are placed in conditions halting this supply. Then we may experience struggle, pain, even terror, as in drowning. Similarly, these other needs are also barely noticeable until we, or circumstances, place us in positions of deprivation. Then it is that physical, mental or emotional pain, or terror, may assert themselves, as in 'nervous breakdown' or depression. For these are the voices of our being telling us of needs, of deprivation. Such a need may be as simple as taking more relaxation, or as complex as unlocking our love, that it may pour into our marriage.

As this book attempts to be a practical one, the question therefore has to be asked: 'How can we recognise our innate needs of body, soul and spirit before they become symptoms of pain?'

Our chapter on diet dealt with general dietary needs; the chapter on postures with general means of satisfying the need for exercise. But we each may have very personal needs. In the practice of relaxation some of these needs may be met. For instance, you may have had too tight a hold on your feelings and the relaxation can release them. Or else tears of grief or loneliness may have been bottled up, and the relaxation allows them expression. Relaxation also is a time of quiet when Life can act upon us and balance our nature, gradually realign emotions and attitudes, and work on us generally in innumerable ways. At such times things we have left undone, such as words of encouragement to a friend, the dropping of anger that has caused conflict between ourselves and another person, a promise unkept, may arise to consciousness to remind us that we cannot find peace, we cannot relax, while such things exist in our life. Sometimes it is like an inner voice, often very real; or an inner realisation of some clarity, that helps us to see our innate needs. Such things occur far more frequently during relaxation simply because our attention is not immersed in outer impressions and activities. Other people have vivid mental pictures or daydreams, often of a symbolical nature, that advise them of their inner nature. These are all means by which Life may express its needs to our awareness. The fact that it sometimes appears as a voice, or pictures, or as a teacher, is simply because of the way the mind works. Just as our feelings may clothe themselves in words when we express them, so these unconscious forces may clothe themselves in images, symbols, colours or words, which arise from within us. This is why dreams are such a helpful way of discovering our inner nature if we go to the trouble of learning their symbolical language.

Thus, in saying that relaxation and peace in life arise from living in harmony with our own complete nature to the best of our capability, we can already begin to see ways of aiding this process. As this book has to keep closely to the aim of dealing only with what can be used with practical advantage by the mother-to-be, I will deal but briefly with what we have covered.

1. *Relaxation.* Having already covered this, nothing more

will be said. For those with a religious temperament, however, prayer, meditation and worship are also means of what we have called 'relaxation'. That is, the way of growing unity between what has caused us to be, and what we are. Whether we call our cause, God, or Source, or Life, or anything else, matters not at all, for it remains what it is whatever we call it or think of it. As the voice said to Moses: 'I am that I am.'

2. *Pain*. Whether this is physical, emotional or mental, it is a signal that something is 'not well' in our being. When it becomes severe physical illness, mental breakdown or emotional agony, we have been misapplying our life for a long period. It is far better to take notice of the little pain than press on regardless towards our own sickness. Pain is a message. Sometimes it is easy to understand if we but stop and listen to it and attempt to see what is causing it. At other times it is more difficult to interpret or understand its meaning, in which case we should seek professional help wherever possible. For the doctor has been trained to interpret the messages of physical pain; and the counsellor or psychiatrist to interpret the emotional and mental ones. For some people these are not their chosen source of help, but at least they should go to their own chosen ones.

3. *Appetites*. These are another way in which our being, physical and mental, announces its needs. In a very real sense the unrest or desire to breathe is an expression of our 'appetite' for air. Appetites express themselves in numerous different ways, announcing needs such as hunger for food, desire for sexual intercourse, thirst for water, tiredness for rest, search for knowledge, longing for love, wanting to play. All these announce needs we must be careful to fulfil, but also careful not to glut. Fortunately, feelings within us quickly tell us what is enough or too much, if we but listen.

4. *The inner voice*. The action of an 'inner voice' becomes far less of a mystery if we but understand something of our own being. Most of us realise for instance that we can only recall a very small part of the information stored in our memory. The other enormous mass of facts, insights, experiences, lessons, nevertheless still exists ready to respond in times of need.

Such response may be subtle, but it is still clear enough if we listen. As an adult we probably cannot remember the first time we burnt our fingers on something hot. But even though we cannot recall the event, or events, the voice of experience still speaks to us clearly through the urge to avoid heat. Similarly, the mass of our experience will talk to us not in a logical process or memory, but as an urge, or seemingly irrational feeling or impulse. While, through our reasoning, we may decide that our car is fit for a long journey, we may have an irrational feeling it is going to break down. If we attempted to listen to this feeling and discover where it has arisen from, we might, for the sake of argument, find that it centres around an engine noise we had not been conscious of before, but now realise indicates a similar fault that caused a breakdown in the past.

Sometimes this intuitive voice becomes so defined in action that it seems as if our total experience actually talks to us. This is undoubtedly the inner voice that Socrates spoke of. Not only does it arise from our total past experience, but also from a contact with the unconscious processes of our being.

If we consider for a moment, there is nothing at all strange about this process of inner guidance or direction. Virtually every moment of the day we are being moved or influenced by subtle feelings of desire for pleasure, security, longing for love, food, comfort, need for assurance, encouragement, urge to know, and so on and on. If you analysed a day's activities, even such simple acts as going out with a friend, going to the toilet, being late for work, choosing a book from the library, you would find all of them were influenced by particular feelings or urges pushing you to comply. It is only because some people train themselves to listen intently to themselves, or have a particular type of make-up, that the voice becomes so clear. If it is mental images we see instead of a voice, these are best understood as dreams due to their often symbolical nature.

It is folly, however, to think of such a voice as an all-seeing oracle. The urges that arise in us may be the voice of our fear, or ambition, or sexual desire. So we have to use some discrimination in deciding whether the voice is representative of our whole being, or just an urge from a split-off energy such as some sexuality is. Also, the voice should only be a guide, never a master. Cautious experiment with following its advice will soon decide its source. For its results are its best judge. 'By their fruits ye shall know them.'

Even so, thousands of ordinary and extraordinary men and women have discovered wise counsel in their own inner voice. It can guide us in every department of our life, from diet to religion, sexual relationship to business details. Examples will be mentioned under 'Dreams'.

5. *Dreams*. All the things I have mentioned above are ways in which we may come to a closer awareness of Life, its wisdom, power *and* love. (As the faculties of our nature emerge from Life, not only intelligence and energy are expressions of its nature, but love also.) In this way we may meet pregnancy, and in fact life, more fully and satisfyingly. Dreams have been used as a means of self-help and self-understanding throughout all known history. They were also used for the same purpose by some branches of yoga. Patanjali, in his *Yoga Aphorisms*, which is one of the accepted yoga classics, mentions them as such.

It is obvious that I cannot go into a lengthy discussion of dreams, but possibly enough can be given to help you understand some of the most useful dreams that occur during pregnancy.

Often, the most immediately practical or useful dreams are in fact easily understood. For instance, during pregnancy my wife dreamed that she should take iron and calcium tablets. There was nothing symbolic about the dream, although many people would overlook it or ignore it. She took the tablets and her health greatly improved. She later dreamed she should do certain of the yoga postures. Again nothing mysterious or symbolic. Again she followed the advice. It is interesting that the birth of the baby took only two hours.

Other women dream that they should eat particular foods, or ease up on certain activities, take a particular vitamin, and so on. In many cases these dreams are not at all symbolical, but straight statements. Other dreams, equally practical, may be slightly or wholly symbolical. Such dreams may still deal with the basis of diet, exercise, rest, work, and so on, but in most cases will probably be concerned with our relationships with others and our own inner condition of emotions, attitudes, or else in some cases how you can best ready yourself as a parent, to bring into the world a beautiful child. Or else who the child is that is being born, and even what sex.

6.

It's All Happening

Am I Pregnant?
With the modern methods of determining pregnancy, such as the urine test, nobody need be in doubt for long, even during the first few days. But if you do not wish to go to this bother, the pregnancy usually announces itself fairly quickly in clinical ways.

The absence of menstruation is often the first sign one has, although by itself this is by no means proof, as many women miss periods for many other reasons. Also, despite being pregnant, a small or short period may occur.

Some women experience morning sickness almost from the first day of conception, which again is a sign, but not a proof. Of course, from the doctor's point of view, the hearing of the baby's heartbeat may alone constitute proof.

Another of the early signs in a healthy woman is breast change. Some women experience this at every menstruation, but it passes. During pregnancy these breast changes remain. The breast becomes fuller in appearance, and becomes tender, especially the nipples. The colour of the skin around the nipple changes, becomes darker, and this area enlarges into a slightly bubbly appearance. After a few months a liquid may be taken from the nipples, called colostrum.

Other changes may be experienced as need for more sleep; inability to eat large meals; strange desires for particular foods; frequency of urination; sudden increase in weight.

The Doctor
It is best to place yourself in the care of your doctor fairly

soon. He or she will examine you, possibly by asking questions as to when your last period was, and so on. Also the examination may include feeling your abdomen with his or her hand. This is to see if any enlargement of the uterus has taken place. The doctor may also examine the vagina for signs of pregnancy, such as a greater supply of blood to the area. No doubt you will be asked for a urine specimen.

Length of Pregnancy

Add seven days to the first day of your last normal menstruation. Then deduct three months, and this will give you the approximate date of a full term pregnancy. Or else add 280 days to the date of conception. Again, this is an approximate date. To save your working it out, 280 days is forty weeks. The average time of conception is about fourteen days after the last normal period. There is little chance of your giving birth on the exact day, as in a survey only four out of a hundred women gave birth on the estimated day.

Quickening

The baby first moves approximately half way through the pregnancy. That is about the twentieth week or just after. This can therefore act as a rough check on your estimated time of conception.

'In Utero'

In recent years a great deal more has been revealed about what the baby does in the womb. Although it is not generally accepted, as given later, there is a fair amount of evidence to show that the baby is very much aware in the womb. The baby does not breathe, gaining its oxygen from the mother's blood, but it does move and rest. If you are observant you will notice that it goes through cycles of activity. Sometimes, much to the amused consternation of 'mum', baby decides to be active just as 'mum' is trying to go to sleep! These movements are very much like those we can see in a newborn baby – a thrusting of arms and legs.

Babies are also now known to often suck their thumbs or

fingers while still unborn. Also, occasionally, to cry, but only when air has in some way entered the uterus.

The Big Day
If you are going into hospital or a nursing home, have your suitcase packed a couple of weeks in advance. If you plan to follow the advice in this book carefully, also have a little purse in which you can place some vitamin C, E and calcium tablets. Take these with you and keep them by you. You will be allowed to have a book and your purse by you until the baby actually arrives.

First Signs
For many women the first sign that birth is about to begin is the breaking of the membranes. Sometimes this happens while asleep in bed, and the resulting puddle of water will undoubtedly wake you. You will have had contractions of the uterus for some weeks. Similar contractions will again appear just prior to, or soon after the water 'breaks', although a few women do not experience the breaking of the membrane.

As soon as the contractions appear however, *right from the start* relax the rest of the body and breathe in stage one as described. Erna Wright points out that if you do not begin the relaxation and breathing right from the beginning the contractions can easily become painful. This is because the contractions are gradually 'opening up' the uterus, and unless the tensions in this area are relaxed, blocking can cause problems from the start.

You may hear the doctor or nurse talking about various stages of labour; to help you understand what they are referring to they are as follows: *First Stage* – The thinning of the 'neck of the uterus' or cervix is a pre-labour stage. The first stage of labour is when the baby's head begins to open up the cervix. This 'opening up' of the cervix is called 'dilating'. The nurse can gradually see more and more of the baby's head as the cervix dilates. She, or the doctor, measures this dilation with finger widths. So she may say 'She's two fingers dilated'. That means that the cervix, which opens rather in the shape of a cat's eye, is two fingers wide. Eventually there is no cervix, only baby's head showing. Then begins the *second stage* of labour, which is when the uterus pushes the baby along the birth channel, *helped now, but not before*, by your abdominal muscles. *The third stage* is after the actual exit of the baby's head and body, and is the removal of the placenta.

What to Do Next
After this quick preview, let us return to the first contractions. As each one occurs, stand still, relax, while breathing in the first stage. From now on your breathing and relaxation is the real thing, not practice. If you feel you must breathe faster to get more air, then do so, as you are not supplying enough. If you breathe out fully each time, this will ensure fuller exchange of air. A feeling of dizziness means you are over-oxygenating. Slow up and do not breathe quite so deeply. On the other hand, trembling is due to a build-up of carbon dioxide in the blood, which is caused by too shallow quick breathing. Take deeper breaths.

If the contractions start during the night, get up if you must, and have a drink of warm milk and honey. But it is better to simply go back to sleep. During this pre-labour phase, contractions may come far apart, or close together, but they are only short in length – ten to twenty seconds. Erna Wright says that the first stage of labour is characterised not so much by frequent contractions as by their length of about forty-five to fifty-five seconds. You must enquire beforehand at which stage your hospital or district nurse wishes to be informed.

Meanwhile, do not tire yourself out during this phase, because you will need all your energy for later on. If it is daytime and you are not requested to enter hospital, then get on with any simple tasks at hand, stopping at each contraction, breathing in level one, and relaxing. From the beginning of the contractions take a 100 mlg of vitamin C every half hour. Carry this on right to the last stage of labour. Also take 1000 i.u. of vitamin E, 4 calcium or 6 kelp tablets and one halibut liver oil capsule at the start of the contractions. Have these all sorted out beforehand so that it is easy. As already said, the C should be continued throughout, one every half hour. The calcium should be taken two every hour. Or if you can't manage that, take 1000 mlg of C at the start and forget about it. The same applies to the calcium.

As the contractions lengthen you will find the level one breathing inadequate. Therefore, shift up into levels two and three as necessary. By the time you reach the 55-second contractions, you should be using the three levels at each contraction. As it begins, say mentally 'contraction beginning', and use level one breathing for 3 breaths, 3 in level 2, the height of the contraction in level 3, and then come down to 3 breaths in two, 3 in one, and say mentally 'contraction finished'.

When the contractions last from one to one-and-a-half minutes, as it begins say mentally, 'contraction beginning', then breathe once in level one, 5 times in level two, the peak of the contraction in level three and then down into level two for 5 breaths and 3 in level one. Then say mentally 'contraction finished'. In between contractions, fully relax, repeating mentally 'surrender to Life'.

The breathing method can be changed to a very fast pant where more air is needed. You can practise this during the last two months of pregnancy with the aid of your husband. With a watch he can time your contractions of arms and legs, and you can practise the breathing routine to get the knack of timing. This will make it all far easier on the day.

I must stress however, that although the above method of breathing at a particular level in each phase of contraction sounds complicated, it very soon becomes a habit if practised often. Quite frankly, you do not have to breathe exactly the number of breaths at each level, as long as you do change as the contraction develops.

What Now?
When your 'waters' do break take a note of the time so that you can inform the nurse or hospital. Doctors who plan to

give their patients a general anaesthetic advise women not to eat before being admitted to hospital. As you are having a natural birth this rule does not apply. The rule is made so that the patient does not vomit stomach contents under anaesthesia and then have the food enter the lungs. Therefore have a small meal to give you sufficient fuel to burn during the activity ahead. As you will not be able to eat for some time, you will need food that will be easy to digest yet will supply a steady flow of fuel. The breakfast already mentioned, which keeps the blood sugar level high for many hours, is excellent for this purpose. That is, a meal consisting mostly of protein, but with carbohydrates, sugars and some fat also. A poached egg on toast, with plenty of butter, followed by a milk drink with a couple of spoonfuls of powdered milk added, plus honey, will be excellent. Or any meal of a similar composition.

Meanwhile, at every contraction except those occurring while you sleep, use the relaxation and breathing technique. Try to get as much sleep as possible before the first stage of labour begins as after this you will have to remain awake and 'working' almost continuously until the end of the labour. To quote Erna Wright, 'Handling contractions during this period is almost like a holy ritual. You handle each contraction with as much single minded concentration and care as you can; in the correct manner, with the correct dissociation, with the correct breathing. Never, *never* answer questions during a contraction.' (*The New Childbirth*). Erna Wright also suggests buying a little, *real* sponge to dip in a saucer of water by the bedside to wipe the face between contractions and to suck for water *and* for comfort. Another helpful tip she gives is to empty the bladder every hour during labour. This is because during labour the usual sensation of a full bladder may not be noticeable. Thus one may reach a point where pain occurs with every contraction due to a full bladder.

Going Great Guns
As stage one of labour changes into stage two after the thinning of the cervix, quite a number of women experience what

is called the *transition stage*. This is experienced as a great tiredness, or feeling of being desperately fed up with the whole process. You may become extremely irritable and bad tempered, but if you can hold on to your discipline for a while, you will pass through this phase. At this time the urge comes to aid the uterus by pushing, using your abdominal muscles, but resist this temptation completely unless the nurse says it is time to push. To help you through this phase if it becomes pronounced enough to disturb you, hold rigidly to your breathing and relaxation discipline, even though these may seem to go haywire for a while, *keep on with them.* Also, every time you relax between contractions say mentally, 'surrender to Life', and completely relax all muscles not in use. As you say this mentally, feel as if you were handing your whole being over, as practised during relaxation, to the light.

Bring On the Reinforcements

You and your uterus are now working full out, but due to your breathing and relaxation you are handling your contractions and they have not become painful. During contractions some women have a cramp-like sensation in the uterus. With your vitamin E and calcium already under your belt, your muscles should perform like trained circus athletes, but just in case, you can rid yourself of this problem. This is done by you, or your husband if he is there, gently and delicately massaging the area in a circular direction. There should be hardly any pressure attached to this, as it is the lightness of touch that soothes the underlying muscles.

Another helpful aid as you enter the second stage of labour is to 'take aim'. In other words, when you actually begin to help the uterus by pushing, it is a great aid to find a spot at the foot of the bed, down beyond the feet, and imagine you are pushing the baby towards it.

Meanwhile, you are still some way from stage three, so don't forget your vitamin C every half-hour, and calcium every hour. If you buy something like Super Rose Hip, or children's flavoured vitamin C tablets, you can suck them like sweets instead of attempting to swallow them.

Erna Wright is so full of practical suggestions it is difficult to avoid quoting her. If it is necessary for the doctor or nurse to examine you internally, or snip the membranes with scissors if they have not been broken, and during the removal of the placenta, Erna suggests that you practise the same rules as for contractions, i.e., go into level two breathing and relax the genitals.

The Birth

Once the cervix has thinned and the baby's head emerges from the vagina, having been pushed along the birth channel, it is usually only a matter of moments before the rest of the baby follows, and you have that wonderful first glimpse of your child.

But before all this occurs, you will be working away at the longest of the contractions, which also require you to 'push' as well. This 'pushing' is the same sort of abdominal tension as that made during going to the toilet. You will have already practised this as advised elsewhere in the book. Make sure, as always, that the genital area is relaxed. As it is difficult to 'push' and breathe at the same time, a slightly different routine is required. In stage two of delivery you will find that as the contraction starts your abdominal muscles will also contract, this contraction is heightened by your own conscious effort. Therefore, as you feel the contractions beginning, say mentally, 'contraction starting', and take three breaths in level two. Then as you breathe in for the fourth time hold your breath in while you push. Hold this for six to ten seconds, depending on your ability, and then blow the air out and repeat. While in the 'pushing' stage, it is best to have plenty of pillows behind you, knees drawn up, back slightly rounded, in imitation of the squat position. As you hold your breath in, push the chin down hard on the chest to block any escape of air, and prevent you arching your head back. As you breathe out, say mentally 'surrender to Life'. Then breathe in again and hold it as above. Repeat this cycle of breathing in, holding it, pushing, blowing out and surrendering, two or three times, depending on length of

contractions. As the contraction begins to wane, no longer
hold the breath, but breathe in level three until you get your
breath back; drop into level two for a few breaths, and then
to level one. Don't forget to relax back *gently* from the
squat position after the contraction so that the baby's head
does not slip back from its position in the birth channel.

As the head of the baby emerges and the rest of the body is
following, no more 'pushing' is necessary. Now is the time to
drop back into the position of sexual surrender, with your own
head dropped back in relaxation, hips and genitals open to
'giving', and mouth open panting as in orgasm.

After the actual birth, the umbilical cord is clipped or tied,
and then severed. The placenta is usually delivered by one
more contraction. Erna Wright suggests, when this is all over,
sucking a few glucose sweets or taking some honey to replace
the blood sugar burnt up during the labour. If you have
already had a previous child you will later experience small
contractions as the uterus returns to its proper size. Handle
these in the same way as you did the birth contractions and
they will soon pass away. The same applies to the contractions
occurring during breast feeding.

Now you should be home and dry. Cuddle baby, forget
everything, and sleep.

7.

Problems

This chapter will deal simply with methods of diet, and exercise, that can be used to cure or minimise some of the problems women face in pregnancy.

Acidity
If little exercise is taken, increase it to include stimulating walks, practising deep breathing as you walk. Increase the amount of raw, 'alkaline' foods, and exclude concentrated starches such as white bread, or white sugar. Do not mix starches and sugar too much in one meal. (See health questionnaire on 'stomach'.) Take at least two dessert-spoons of brewer's yeast powder daily. Use the apple fast if necessary, as it is a very quick cure. Much acidity or indigestion is caused by inner tensions, and the relaxation and 'earthquake' posture should be used frequently.

Age
If you are an elderly mother, check your health carefully against the health questionnaire, and follow directions. It is best to start with very high doses of the vitamins and minerals, and drop them week by week to the 'under par' dosage given in Chapter 3, No 11 under 'Full Diet' (page 71). Therefore start with 1,000 i.u. of vitamin C, the same with vitamin E;* halibut oil capsules as directed on the bottle; 4 dessert-spoons of brewer's yeast and wheatgerm; and a multi-vitamin and mineral supplement daily for one week, 800 i.u. of vita-

* Vitamin E should not be used in higher doses than 400 i.u. per day if suffering from high blood-pressure or a rheumatic heart condition.

min C and 800 i.u. of E for the second week, and from the third week drop the C and E by 100 units per week until you reach the 'under par' dosage as given in the chapter just mentioned.

Alcoholism

If the mother is an alcoholic it is possible to bring about marked changes in health, and reduce if not remove the need for alcohol. Adelle Davis gives the following suggestions that have been tried with great success at a 'home' for alcoholics. Six small high-protein meals per day, free of all refined carbohydrates, are taken. This includes plenty of lean meat, eggs, fish, milk with dried milk added, yogurt, and brewer's yeast, which, weight for weight, has more protein than other foods, and fulfils dietary needs in an alcoholic. Also, high doses of lecithin, calcium and magnesium, taken as halibut oil capsules, backed by multivitamin and mineral capsules. This should also be used with the raw food diet where possible. It is the B vitamins that are particularly needed, thus brewer's yeast, and B-complex tablets should also be used. Alcohol destroys many vitamins in the system, thus these recommendations. Slow breathing should be practised daily. *See also* **Depression.**

Allergies

Hay fever, asthma, and many other allergies are often greatly reduced or cured by enormous doses of vitamin C. 2,000 i.u. daily is indicated, until the attack has been cured. If high C intake causes looseness of the bowels, start at a low dosage and work up.

Anaemia

As many raw green leaves as possible, including dandelion, watercress, cress, sprouts, kale, broccoli, lettuce, peppers, etc., should be eaten. Also daily take plenty of brewer's yeast, 400 i.u. of vitamin E, one vitamin and mineral capsule daily, with vitamin B_{12} as suggested on the bottle. Also the 'Full Diet' (page 69), with added wheatgerm.

Ankles, swollen

There can be several causes of this, and each should be checked. The foremost is constipation or sluggish bowel, delivering hard stools. See the suggestions under 'Intestines' in the health questionnaire. Balanced diet, with plenty of raw foods, with carrageen moss beaten into milk, and wheatgerm, will help or cure the hard stools. Other possible causes are insufficient protein in the diet, or too much salt. A protein deficiency can be filled by beating dried milk, or lecithin powder, into one's milk drink, or added to cereals, and taking plenty of brewer's yeast. It is important to get plenty of raw foods and green leaves also. Another factor may be lack of vitamin F, or unsaturated fatty acids. Strangely enough, one needs such oils to keep slim and lose weight due to water retention. Therefore, if you can see that inadequate vegetable oils, as from nuts, maize, wheatgerm, and sunflower seeds, are included in the diet, remedy this and also add some olive oil, safflower oil, or wheatgerm oil to one's daily foods.

Birth

An easy delivery is aided by taking raspberry leaf tea, or tablets, throughout pregnancy. High doses of vitamins C and E during labour will greatly enhance the effectiveness of the raspberry leaf tablets. That is, at the commencement of labour take 1,000 i.u. of E and 1000 mg. of C. Make sure that calcium tablets are taken during the last week, and four at the beginning of labour, as this alone has resulted in painless births. The calcium should contain vitamin D.

Blood-pressure

Very often caused by a too high salt intake. Dr Dahl, in experiments, has shown that high blood-pressure in babies has resulted from feeding tinned baby food, which contains high amounts of salt. High blood-pressure can also be caused by a cholin deficiency, which can be reduced by either taking cholin, or brewer's yeast.

Low blood-pressure may indicate insufficient protein intake.

Breath, shortness of
Apart from the pressure on the diaphragm near the end of
term, this can indicate lack of B vitamins, to be found in
brewer's yeast, and anaemia. The exercises and breathing
practices will also help.

Constipation
It is not true that constipation is natural during pregnancy.
It is widespread – but not natural. It can result from lack of
raw foods, and insufficient whole cereal grains or wholewheat
flour in the diet. It can, in many cases, be immediately cured
by a few slices of wholewheat bread daily. Whole wheat must
not be confused with 'brown bread' or wholemeal, which are
quite different. Brewer's yeast, wheatgerm, and carrageen
moss beaten into milk will all help remove this condition.
Some people find a few bananas daily aids the problem. In
difficult cases, bran should be taken, and multi-vitamin and
mineral tablets might help.

Cramps
These should not occur if you are eating the Full Diet as given
(page 69), with supplements. This condition is basically due to
insufficient calcium or magnesium in the diet; but also links
up with B vitamins, as in brewer's yeast, and vitamin D. If the
supplements as suggested are being taken, it is most likely
that the calcium and magnesium are insufficient. Extra
calcium should be taken, either as kelp or bone-meal or
straight calcium tablets, with one multi-vitamin and mineral
tablet.

Dandruff
If this develops during pregnancy it is a sign that you have
become deficient in vitamin A and B and need more fruit.
However, if the suggested diet and supplements have been
taken, there should be no sign of this. As some people have
greater needs for particular vitamins, it might suggest a need
for more vitamin A with the supplements. Extra halibut oil
capsules should help.

Depression

Here is another common, although often unnecessary, aspect of child-bearing, and sometimes even after birth. If this happens despite following the dull diet and supplements, it is suggested you regularly practise slow breathing. To do this, sit quietly and breathe as slowly as possible without having to gasp. Try to breathe smoothly as well as slowly. Practise for ten minutes every day, and gradually increase the time to half an hour.

Diarrhoea

If diarrhoea continues for more than a day, it can be dangerous due to flushing out necessary nutrients. Rest, and apples or carrots (raw) only, will quickly cure. The first meal should consist of milk, slippery elm food, and carrageen moss (1 teaspoon) mixed into a cream, with honey. Do not keep eating mixed diet if it continues for longer than twenty-four hours, but eat only apples or carrots plus garlic tablets.

Drug addiction

See **Alcoholism.**

Edema

See **Ankles.**

Epilepsy

Dolomite tablets, and sometimes Epsom salts, due to their high magnesium content, can often completely remove convulsions, and as long as sufficient magnesium is taken in a balanced diet, they will not return. Convulsions in babies will often respond similarly. Vitamin B_6 is also used to control convulsions.

Fatigue

Excessive fatigue is often due to a badly balanced diet, high in sweets, sugar, carbohydrates, and low in proteins, vitamins and minerals. Often such people miss breakfast, eat sweets, drink strong tea or coffee. Anaemia and low blood-pressure are also factors to be taken into account. In such cases it is wise to eat an egg, and have a milk drink fortified with dried milk, for breakfast, as well as balancing the diet as given in the 'Full Diet' (page 69). See the breakfast recommended in the 'Weight-losing Diet', page 68. Incorrect breathing may also be the cause. See Chapter 4 on breathing.

Fertility

In cases where couples are unable to have children it is suggested that both go on an apple fast for three days. See the 'Cleansing Diet' on page 65. This should be followed by coming back to the 'Full Diet' (page 69), with the following supplements: 300 mlg of vitamins E and C per day, and the other supplements suggested under No. 11 under the 'Full Diet', page 71. If there is a tendency to catarrh, garlic tablets should be taken; they leave no odour.

No attempt should be made to conceive until a full month on these supplements and diet has passed. Also, if in going through the health questionnaire other things are indicated, these should be taken also. Once conception has taken place, the basic diet and supplements for pregnancy should be taken. It is helpful to add wheatgerm to the diet also. The father's diet is as important, prior to conception, as the mother's.

How long may conception take on this diet? This is impossible to predict. Benjamin Sieve, M.D., experimented with a group of twenty-two women who had remained childless for at least five years. His only addition to their diet was PABA, a part of the B vitamin group, and found in brewer's yeast. The result was that twelve of the group bore healthy babies within two years.

The above diet programme attempts to hit more of the possible causes of childlessness than PABA deficiency. Therefore, please attempt to follow it fully. With all the dietary modifications a year should be long enough in most cases to see, one way or the other, whether conception will take place under these methods. Sufficient exercise must also be taken. In other words, an effort must be made to attain positive good health.

Flatulence
If this is painful, or really bad smelling, it is very often caused by an unbalanced diet, insufficient intestinal bacteria, digestive enzymes, hydrochloric acid and B vitamins. This ties up strongly with the condition of one's tongue. If the tongue is always coated, or if it is sore, or deep red or magenta, or if the edges are scalloped, or if there are deep fissures in it, or if the taste buds are much enlarged or un-evenly distributed, or if it is too large or too small a tongue; these all show signs of vitamin B deficiencies, and enzyme, acid, or bacterial imbalance. If adequate B vitamins, in the form of yeast, wholewheat flour, and wheatgerm are being taken, it is suggested that for a week or two, hydrochloric acid tablets and digestive enzyme tablets be taken, along with two multi-vitamin and mineral tablets daily. The flatulence should stop in a day or two if you have hit the cause. In this case continue until the flatulence does not occur, and the tongue clears up. Plenty of brewer's yeast powder should be taken, along with liver, calcium tablets, and dates. I have found eating only yogurt for two days very helpful in such cases. As much can be eaten as wished.

Fluoridation
Many nutritionists look upon artificial fluoridation of water as a drug. As medical opinion is against drug use during pregnancy, it should also be against water fluoridation. Animal research has shown that fluorides cause the dis-solving of the forming heart tissue in the embryo. Carlton Frederick, in *Food Facts and Fallacies*, says, 'Significantly, the rate of the birth of stillborn babies in New Britain, Connecticut, went up 150 per cent after fluoridation. The rate in adjacent communities without fluoridation did not change in that period. Studies have also shown a higher incidence of mongoloid births in fluoridated water areas.'
Other research has proved that harmful fluorides, or in

fact many poisons, are 'floated' out of the system by vitamin C when taken in sufficient quantities. Therefore, if you live in an area where the water is fluoridated, 300 mlg of vitamin C daily will act as a preventative measure.

Hay fever
See **Allergies**

Headaches
If the diet is already sufficient in the way described, and headaches have only begun with pregnancy, it is possibly a sign of calcium lack. Even migraines can often be eradicated by sufficient calcium and magnesium where the diet is otherwise sufficient, especially in the B vitamins.

Heart
If the prospective mother has a heart condition, 600 i.u. of vitamin E should be taken daily throughout pregnancy, with the other basic supplements, and the wholefood diet. Many heart conditions are literally cured by this treatment, but at the least it will take much strain off the heart. As magnesium has also cured many heart conditions, a quarter teaspoon of Epsom salt daily is a wise precaution, as it is a muscle food.

Hot flushes
These, like headaches, where the diet is otherwise sufficient, often indicate a deficiency in calcium and magnesium.

Infertility
See **Fertility.**

Insomnia
This may point to a greater need of the B vitamins in yeast, and to calcium lack. Practising the relaxation techniques will help in this problem, and de-tensing the body while in bed often aids sleep. The slow breathing technique already described under 'Depression' is also an enormous help, especially if used just prior to sleep.

Labour

To make labour easy, raspberry leaf tea or tablets should be taken throughout pregnancy. I have known women who have used them produce their baby in half an hour or two hours. Also, stress is reduced by taking 1000 i.u. of vitamin E as labour commences, and 100 mlg of vitamin C every half-hour. Pain is reduced or removed by taking four calcium tablets with vitamin D as labour starts, and one every hour. Adelle Davis quotes some mothers who have used calcium tablets and vitamin D in this way, as saying that they thought they were only having wind pains when the baby was born. It would be even more effective to take the extra calcium and D during the whole of the last week. *See also* **Birth.**

Legs, swelling of
See **Ankles.**

Miscarriage

Where there is not a physical cause for miscarriage such as fibroid tumour in the uterus, tears in the cervix, malformation of reproductive organs, high blood-pressure, diabetes, or syphilis, the general state of health is often the reason. Many women who miscarry can have a successful pregnancy once their general health and nutrition is taken care of. Even regular miscarriages can frequently be avoided by sensible diet, exercise and rest.

This book may come into the hands of women at all stages of pregnancy, and even prior to conception. It is obviously best to begin one's health renovation prior to conception, but I have seen an advanced pregnancy that medically seemed ripe for miscarriage, yet responded immediately when supplements and raw foods were added to the diet.

Therefore, if you have a history of miscarriage, and have not conceived, but plan to, I would suggest that husband and wife should start with the cleansing diet, whichever version is acceptable, although I would recommend the apple diet. Come back on to the 'Full Diet' (page 69), with the following supplements and dietary additions. For the husband,

100 i.u. of vitamin E daily, with a multi-vitamin and mineral capsule. For the wife, flood the body with vitamin C for a week by taking 2000 mlg per day. It may be best to work up to this dose over a few days. Drop the dose to 300 per day throughout conception and pregnancy, after this one week at 2000 mlg. Vitamin C strengthens the capillaries, and thus aids the strength and health of the placenta and baby. For the first week, 1000 i.u. of vitamin E per day, and then drop to 300 i.u. per day throughout conception and pregnancy. Take the other supplements as in No. 11 under 'Full Diet' (page 71). If possible, get vitamin C and E tablets that contain the whole vitamins.

Go through the health questionnaire and see whether there are any other needs, in which case (as with poor skin needing extra vitamin A) fulfil the need. Eat as many oranges as are enjoyable each day. Be careful in peeling them to leave as *much of the white pith on* as possible. The pith of the orange contains what are called bio-flavonoids, which are very necessary to the health of the placenta. Vitamin K likewise, when deficient, compensates to miscarriage. This is found in green leaves such as raw cabbage, kale, carrot greens, spinach; also in tomatoes, egg yolk, cauliflower, and liver.

Anaemia is a contributory cause of miscarriage, but if the Full Diet is followed this should be under control. If there is still anaemia, take 'Iron Plus' tablets. These contain vitamin C, aiding its digestion, and making the tablet less constipating.

Other additions to the diet should be 4 dessertspoons of wheatgerm daily, and black treacle or molasses used in making any cakes, bread or puddings.

If you are already pregnant, take the supplements as described (i.e., a large dose to start), and begin the other dietary suggestions as far as possible. I realise that many people are temperamentally against salads and some of the other suggested foods. But all that is asked is to follow them as far as possible, and I know that many will then have a successful pregnancy and a beautiful baby.

For those women already pregnant, and who are suffering

a threatened miscarriage, Dr Shute of Canada holds out a great deal of hope. It is common medical philosophy that a spontaneous miscarriage usually means that the foetus is possibly unhealthy or malformed, and the body is trying to be rid of it. Dr Shute did not accept this attitude, but felt that while this may hold true in a very few cases, the majority of miscarriages are due to factors of nutrition causing an unhealthy placenta. In working with several hundred women, using 100 to 400 mlg of vitamin E daily, he was able to cause virtually all of the threatened miscarriages to revert to a state of health, and result in the birth of healthy babies. Therefore, in such cases, it will be wise to go on to the Full Diet, with the suggested supplements as given above, i.e., 500 mlg of vitamin C, 300 of vitamin E, with brewer's yeast, kelp and wheatgerm.

Morning sickness
I have noticed that women who are suffering from morning sickness, and then go on to the vitamin mineral supplements, often lose their sickness very quickly. Carlton Frederick says, 'If the diet and the use of supplements are instituted prior to pregnancy, the incidence of morning sickness may be sharply diminished.' Research has shown that vitamin B_6 plays a large part in curing or preventing this sickness. Therefore, brewer's yeast should be taken in ample quantities, and if necessary a B_6 supplement. Fairly large amounts of B_6 may be necessary to *cure* the sickness, but little to prevent it.

A further aid is given by Bircher Benner. He suggests a few raisins, pine kernels and mint leaves eaten on waking. Also dry wholewheat bread, with cream cheese, nuts, fruit and dried fruit for breakfast. A helpful general rule is to eat a small snack on waking. This is something found most helpful if very dry, such as toasted wholewheat bread. The succeeding meals should be small but often, five or six per day are suggested, and eating just a few things each meal. That is, few mixtures.

Nerves
See Depression.

Neuralgia
Use the apple fast or cleansing akaline diet. The results are
dramatic.

Oral contraceptives
If they have been used, this increases the need for the B
vitamins, and vitamin E.

Piles
See 'Intestines' in the health questionnaire (page 59).

Poisoning
Poisons, such as lead, bromide, arsenic, benzine, fluorides,
ivy, some snake bites, or insect bites, gas or car fumes, can be
removed by massive doses of vitamin C. 3000 mlg each day,
for one week, should be taken. Vitamin E has a similar
power, so 300 i.u. should be taken with the vitamin C.

Prenatal
In breast-feeding the baby, one should check to see that the
diet is sufficient, especially in vitamins A, D, C, and E, and
calcium. Formulas are not recommended by nutritionists,
nor for the emotional health of the baby.

Prolapse
Prolapse during pregnancy can be very painful, and is experienced as sharp pains in the groin, or sometimes as severe
backache. This can be cured or greatly relieved by taking
from 300 to 600 i.u. of vitamin E daily. Experiment on the
low dose to see if it works; if not, increase. Also increase the
calcium intake.

Pyorrhoea
If this develops while pregnant, it shows a greater need for
vitamins B, C, and D; C in particular.

Salivation

Excess salivation can be helped by eating very dry meals. Going on the cleansing diet for a few days will be of great help also. It is not recommended to do the apple diet for more than one day if pregnant, but the other cleansing diet is safe for up to a week. A very dry mouth sometimes accompanies vitamin A deficiency.

Sciatica
See **Neuralgia.**

Sterility
See **Fertility.**

Varicose veins

These can usually be avoided by taking care to watch bowel action. If the stools become slightly hard, add more carrageen moss to drinks, and wheatgerm and brewer's yeast to the diet. If this is insufficient, bran will usually help. But the stools must be consistently soft at each passing. If you are on the full diet and supplements, this will go a long way to preventing this. 400 mlg of vitamins C and E daily will help if the stools are soft. Sometimes cramps and varicosities occur together. In this case, besides the vitamin E, take a B complex tablet. *See also* Constipation.

Vaginal discharge

If very heavy and thick, may point to a vitamin A need, as this vitamin helps control the health of all mucous membrane. Also, a more alkaline diet will help to clean the body.

Weight

It has often happened in my experience that people put on an adequate diet lose or gain weight to become a normal weight. If the Full Diet here suggested (page 69) is followed, the person should find little excess of weight gain. The daily salad is important in this respect. Causes of excess weight gain can be due to insufficient iodine and vitamin E in the diet. These are found in kelp tablets and wheatgerm. It may also be caused by a lack of protein, thus causing water retention, as does excess salt in the diet. One can easily boost protein intake by taking extra eggs, yogurt or yeast daily. Insufficient vegetable oils such as safflower, olive oil, etc., may have a similar result.

Obviously, if you are not on the Full Diet as suggested, it could be that you are simply eating far too many sugar and flour products.

As a postscript to this section, an enormous amount of information concerning baby care has arisen in recent years. Love has at last come into its own as a scientifically observable healing agent. It is now acknowledged that the newborn baby often has the instinct to immediately suckle, and needs to be held close and lovingly, if possible skin to skin, as soon as born. Looking into your baby's eyes, holding, cuddling, playing and caressing, are all expressions of love, and the baby needs it as much as food. It has even been shown that babies who are loved and caressed often, especially skin to skin, are less prone to infection than babies seldom handled or rocked.

8.

Childlessness

Looking at the conditions of some women who have been unable to have children, and who have never adopted any, one can see childlessness can have an extraordinary influence. The women may become prone to excessive worry and nervousness, compulsive talking, health fears, owners of pampered dogs, and cut off from deep contact with others. Just as the lack of fulfilment in the sexual instinct can cause frustration and neurotic symptoms, so does the lack of fulfilment of the mothering instinct in some women cause similar conditions. A man or woman may find an acceptable means of expressing and fulfilling the emotions and energies that lie behind the sexual urge, other than in sexual intercourse. Likewise, some women express their tenderness and need to care and cherish in other ways than raising a baby. However, it is not only women who feel urged to parenthood. Many men also have very great inner drives to produce a baby.

Nevertheless, this chapter is more concerned with ways and means the childless couple can use to overcome their barrenness. Despite the fact that hope can be held out to a number of such couples, it is none the less a difficult subject to approach, this being due to the fact that there are so many possible causes of barrenness. Estimates show that one in ten couples in the U.S. are unable to have children. Also, age has a great bearing on it. Before the age of 20, only 4 per cent of women remain childless. From 20 to 24, 6 per cent, 25 to 29, 10 per cent, 30 to 34, 16 per cent.

One of the basic causes, even according to medical opinion, is poor health. Dr Guttmacher says that sound health enhances fertility, and the fertility level of a couple can often be improved to the point where pregnancy will occur by improving nutrition, reducing the overweight and building up the underweight, relieving anaemia, changing conditions that may be causing fatigue or correcting glandular disturbance.

He goes on to say that any means of relieving nervous tension may work miracles.

Other causes can be mumps in male testicles, abdominal surgery, gonorrhea, method of intercourse, sperm content, blocked fallopian tubes, or blocked tubules in the male, over-acidity in the female sex organ, lack of ovulation, thyroid problems, and too many others to list.

What are the practical things to do then?

1. *Health.* Be frank, are you in good health? Do you have much catarrh? In the woman, this rubbish in the system can block the passage in the sex organs, where the sperm should pass. Are you overweight, anaemic, generally depleted, over-worked, on a poor diet high in starches, alcohol, and manu-factured foods? Do you smoke too much? Even if *you* think you are healthy, your childlessness at least questions this. In your diet, exercise and rest, make sure you are more than adequate. Diet and exercise are dealt with more fully in other chapters. Sidney Rose-Neil, a well known naturopath, told me that of the women who come to him for treatment for childlessness nearly all of them are anaemic, and respond to diet therapy.

2. *The sex act.* Do you realise that the most fertile time for the woman is around the fourteenth day after the last period? If so, does intercourse coincide with this? Yoga sees the sex act as something far deeper than most medical philosophy, although the act itself is enough to precipitate pregnancy in most people. If it is directed by love and respect for each other, and climaxed by full orgasm, the results are inwardly different from the unfeeling sex act. We have already seen that nervous tension or psychological problems may cause barren-ness. As the sexual act can be used as the barometer of one's psychological health, it is worth looking more closely at it. For one's inner tensions, fears, guilts or phobias may be

reflected in the sex act. Reich says that full orgasm is the 'capacity for surrender to the flow of biological energy without any inhibition'. This results in *involuntary* pleasurable contractions of the body.

The typical course of fulfilling sexual intercourse he describes as first a pleasurable erection. In cases of long abstinence, premature ejaculation usually occurs, before proper orgasm can be achieved. Then in the male there is the urge to penetrate; in the female a desire to be penetrated. The man is naturally gentle through feelings of love, and not because he is covering up feelings of aggressiveness, sadism, or desires to bite or hurt. The woman feels she is drawing the man in, the man, that he is being drawn in. In the disturbed emotions, this may cause tensions or problems. From here the pleasure is intense, without causing rapid ejaculation. The movements become spontaneous, and should be allowed to occur outside of one's conscious will. This calls for an ability to surrender entirely, and talking or laughing show serious lack of surrender. Just as the heart beats without our conscious effort, so the movements of one's body at this time occur even though one has completely 'let go'. Now the pleasure, which was concentrated on and in the sexual organs, begins to spread to the whole body.

Then a sudden increase in excitation occurs. While one could have interfered with the spontaneous movements before, now it becomes impossible. Contractions of the whole pelvis occurs, with a wonderful melting feeling, and there is a tremendous relief of tension. During this there are spontaneous deep breaths or cries of pleasure, the head goes back, the mouth drops open as the orgasm is reached. This is followed by complete relaxation, without any feelings of guilt, disgust, hate, leaden exhaustion, repulsion or indifference. Rather there is a feeling of tenderness and desire to sleep. Only in disturbed satisfaction is there further desire for intercourse.

If this pattern is seriously disturbed, it is worth seeking advice from marriage guidance councillors, or a psychiatrist. Although one *must not* alight on this as *the* cause of barrenness. Many extremely sexually disturbed people have babies.

I have mentioned it only as a possible clue to those whose childlessness is thought to be psychological.

Other causes of barrenness in the sex act may be too frequent or too infrequent intercourse. For those whose sperm count is low, a lapse of some time prior to the fertile period will help the sperm count increase. For those who only have intercourse very occasionally, the sperm ready to emerge sometimes lose their potency, and the second intercourse will contain more active sperm. Similarly, very hot baths, or some drugs, tend to kill the sperm. A hot bath, even some days prior to intercourse, could mean an inactive batch of sperm. Certainly baths should only be comfortably hot. Smoking sometimes does the same thing. Vitamin E helps such conditions enormously.

Intercourse when one is tired also seems to be a cause of barrenness. It is best to wake in the early morning after some hours of sleep, and love each other, then sleep again until it is time to rise.

3. *Dreams*. Take notice of any dreams that suggest changes in diet, mental outlook, or habits.

4. *Medical help*. If none of the above things seem applicable, arrange an appointment at a clinic where thorough examination of both partners can be given. Do not be put off by one's ordinary doctor. I have known such a doctor tell a woman to forget about it and go and buy some new clothes!

Index

Also available from Sphere Books

A BEGINNER'S GUIDE TO YOGA
Nancy Phelan

Facts About Yoga/How Yoga Works/Practising at Home/ Hatha Yoga in the Form of a Lesson/Further Practise/ Mental Training/The Method Plus Yourself/Yoga and Diet/More About Yoga/Practise Guide.

0 7221 6837 3   Fully Illustrated   75p

YOGA OVER FORTY
Michael Volin & Nancy Phelan

Discard the conventional attitude to age!
Dismiss the thought 'Too Old!'
To the practitioner of yoga, the physical body does not stop developing until the age of 33. For him or her 45 is literally 'the prime of life'. This is the message of YOGA OVER FORTY, a complete philosophy by which the middle-aged can, physically and mentally, ensure against the tragedy of increasing ill-health and failing powers.

0 7221 8760 2   Fully Illustrated   65p

All Sphere Books are available at your bookshop or newsagent, or can be ordered from the following address:
Sphere Books, Cash Sales Department,
P.O. Box 11, Falmouth, Cornwall.

Please send cheque or postal order (no currency), and allow 19p for postage and packing for the first book plus 9p per copy for each additional book ordered up to a maximum charge of 73p in U.K.

Customers in Eire and B.F.P.O. please allow 19p for postage and packing for the first book plus 9p per copy for the next 6 books, thereafter 3p per book.

Overseas customers please allow 20p for postage and packing for the first book and 10p per copy for each additional book.